SECOND EDITION

Fundamental Skills in the Nurse-Patient Relationship
a programed text

LIANNE S. MERCER, R.N., B.S.N., M.S.
Clinical Instructor in Psychiatric Nursing,
San Jacinto College, Pasadena, Texas;
formerly Assistant Professor of Nursing,
School of Nursing, The University of Michigan

PATRICIA O'CONNOR, Ph.D.
Senior Research Associate,
Department of Educational Resources,
School of Dentistry, The University of Michigan

W. B. SAUNDERS COMPANY • Philadelphia • London • Toronto

W. B. Saunders Company: West Washington Square
Philadelphia, Pa. 19105

12 Dyott Street
London, WCIA 1DB

833 Oxford Street
Toronto, Ontario M8Z 5T9, Canada

Fundamental Skills in the Nurse-Patient Relationship   ISBN   0-7216-6266-8
A Programed Text

Last digit is the print number: 9   8   7   6   5   4   3   2

To B.J.H.

TO THE INSTRUCTOR

Nursing educators assign great importance to the student's relationships with her patients. However, there are inherent difficulties in providing instruction in this area. Typically, students begin working with patients before the nature of the nurse-patient relationship has been explored in depth. Furthermore, to develop implications for action from principles may be difficult for the instructor and even more difficult for the student. In this programed text we have attempted to offer guidelines for action that students may apply to a wide variety of situations. The program is designed to teach a basic repertoire of skills with which a student may begin her nursing practice.

The beginning nursing student working with patients in the hospital is presented with many situations to which she must respond. For example: What should she say if a patient refuses an ordered treatment? How should she respond when a patient asks questions about his diagnosis or prognosis? How can she acquire information from written resources and from the patient himself when further information is required for action? It is not surprising if the student cannot effectively answer these and other questions or if she feels inadequate when they arise. In this text we have attempted to increase the student's competence and confidence. To achieve these ends we have identified situations that may occur and have shown how they may be approached. Although rationales for action are invariably delineated, the ultimate goal for the program is to enhance the student's competence in the interpersonal aspects of nursing care.

It should be noted that the text is not intended to be a comprehensive treatment of the nurse-patient relationship. It is rather an eight to ten hour instructional unit designed for students who are beginning to work in the hospital setting and who want to develop skills that will serve them well in relating to patients.

We would like to direct your attention to Appendix B which includes the Criterion Test and to the program objectives which preface each instructional sequence designed to teach students to meet the objectives. The objectives and the corresponding test items were written first and only then were the instructional materials developed to teach students to attain each objective as defined by the Criterion Test items. An Instructor's Manual available to all faculty using the programed text includes a key to the examination and suggested weightings for items. In our view, the learning experience of the student will be substantially enhanced if the test is used in the course and if students are given the results of their tests. The Manual also includes the rationale for the program and student performance data.

L. Mercer

P. O'Connor

TO THE STUDENT

This programed text is designed to help you learn fundamental skills in your relationships with your patients. The emphasis is on behavior, i.e., what you should say and do under a variety of conditions in the hospital. For example:

1. How should you introduce yourself to your patients?
2. What should you say to a patient before beginning a treatment?
3. How can you utilize resource information in caring for patients?
4. What should you say when patients ask diagnostic questions about themselves? About others?
5. How may you respond to patients' criticisms of yourself or of the hospital?
6. What should you do when a patient refuses an ordered treatment?
7. When is it necessary to gain more information before taking action? How may information be elicited from patients?
8. How can you encourage patient communication?
9. How can you respond effectively when patients express feelings?
10. How can you assist the patient's efforts in the process of problem solving?
11. How can you evaluate the effect you have in your interactions with patients?

If you are like most students beginning nursing studies, you are not yet able to answer most or all of these questions. After you have completed the program, you will be able to deal with them all effectively.

Although the relationship with patients is the most rewarding facet of nursing for many students, beginning to function as a professional person in relation to others presents a challenge. Typically, students start working in the hospital at about the same time that they begin formal class work. In order to safeguard patients' welfare and maximize student learning, instructors sequence classroom learning and clinical assignments so that students are asked to demonstrate in the hospital skills they have learned in the classroom or laboratory. For example, injections are prepared and administered, dressings changed, and equipment operated only when the instructor believes the student can perform effectively.

The situation is intrinsically different in the student's relationship to the patient. The patient rather than the instructor may pose questions or define the problem. He or she may ask questions about his or her illness, about dietary and activity restrictions, or in fact about anything at all. The patient may seek in the student an understanding listener or a person with whom problems can be worked through. The student must respond.

Later in nursing studies, there will be formal class work in communication skills and in psychiatric nursing. There will be discussions of students' experiences with their own patients. Basic concepts such as conflict, frustration, and anxiety will be developed and applied to nursing care. Students may write verbatim reports of their interactions with patients and analyze the intent and effectiveness of their efforts, but all this will take place later on. In early contacts with patients, students have been "on their own." This text has been written to change this. It attempts to provide students with some basic guidelines which will make them more effective and more confident in dealing with patients.

In order to simulate what actually happens in the hospital setting, we have presented many examples of nurses interacting with patients. Throughout the text you will be given situations and asked to write down what you would say and what action you would take. This is to encourage you to begin to respond on paper as you will in a real situation. Correct answers are provided so that you may check your answers as you go along. This "feedback" will help you to perform well on the examination or, more important, in the clinical setting. Tear off the perforated "slider" attached to the back cover of the book and use it to mask the printed answers until you have written out your own answers. A list of abbreviations and their meanings in the Glossary on page 149 may be consulted when you wish.

This program has been designed to teach students to reach specific behavioral objectives. The Criterion Test in Appendix B was constructed so that each item corresponds to one or more of these objectives. If you answer a question correctly, you will demonstrate that you have met the objective; if you answer all questions correctly you will have met the goals of the program. For your guidance, each objective appears in the program immediately preceding the frames which are directed toward the attainment of the objective.

Frequently in the text, you will be asked to state what you would say to the patient in some particular situation. Obviously, when the "correct" answer is given only one or two direct quotes may be given. Your answer may not be identical to the answers in the program. It should, however, be consistent with the principle exemplified by the answers given in the text. In other words, we have attempted to offer guidelines for actions with examples of correct responses, not passwords, slogans, or set phrases.

A final point about the program should be made. It does not attempt to teach all there is to know about the nurse-patient relationship. For example, very little has been said about non-verbal communication because of the limitations of the printed page. We have not developed in depth some of the basic concepts that would be covered in nursing courses, e.g., frustration, anxiety, and experiential learning. The text does, however, offer a foundation for later learning as well as provide guidelines for the beginning nursing student who wants to know what to say and do in a wide variety of situations.

L. Mercer

P. O'Connor

ACKNOWLEDGMENTS

The development and writing of the first edition of this programed text was supported by the United States Public Health Service in a Project Grant for Improvement in Nurse Training (BSS-NPG 95). We are very grateful for this support.

We would like to acknowledge with thanks the help and encouragement of the faculty and students of the Fundamentals of Nursing course at the University of Michigan. In 1967 and 1968, sophomore students served as test subjects for initial versions of the program and also evaluated the text and made suggestions for change. Performance and opinion data are reflected in this final form.

Barbara Horn was a valuable consultant from the beginning to the conclusion of the project. Her personal commitment to instructional improvement and her enthusiastic support of faculty efforts to bring it about created an ideal environment for our efforts.

Alice Marsden contributed many basic ideas represented in the program and was a helpful consultant throughout the project. Rae Okamoto Yoshida, who served as project director during the first year of the grant, identified and defined the *behaviors* that represent fundamental skills in what proved to be a difficult and amorphous content area. Phyllis Nicolaou gave many vital suggestions while the program was being written and revised and offered not only criticisms but also insights for improvement. Many other faculty members provided useful ideas and support at all stages of the project.

Mrs. Mercer wishes to thank her husband, Charles, for his support and understanding during the preparation of the second edition, and her children, Michelle and Steven, for their lively interest in their mother's work and their perceptive ability to stay out of the way at critical times.

TABLE OF CONTENTS

Part I

_____

UTILIZING RESOURCES IN PATIENT CARE

Utilizing patient resource materials, the student extracts information to answer questions about the patient and correctly draws inferences for nursing action. (Frames 1-38)

Utilizing patient resource materials, the student identifies important questions she should ask the patient and important observations she should make. (Frames 1-38)

1

When the nurse goes into the patient's room, she should know:
 1. The patient's diagnosis and operation, if any.
 2. What treatments are ordered for the patient.
 3. What restrictions the physician has placed on the patient's activities and diet.
 4. What appointments are scheduled for the patient, and at what time.
 5. Whether his oral intake and urinary output are to be measured.
 6. What the patient's condition has been during the past few hours.
 7. The patient's preferences regarding his care in the hospital.
This information will assist the nurse to give effective and individualized care to the patient.

(Go on to the next frame.)

2

You, the nurse, are assigned to care for Mr. Holmes. You have the following questions about your care for him. Suppose that you begin care for him without the answers to any of these questions, how effective would your care be?
 1. What is his diagnosis?
 2. What treatments are scheduled?
 3. How many times a day should each treatment be done and, where appropriate, for how long?
 4. How does he prefer that they be done?
 5. What appointments are scheduled? At what time? What preparation is necessary?
 6. What are his activity limitations and specifically prescribed activities?
 7. What medications are ordered? At what time?
 8. Is it necessary to measure intake and output? What was yesterday's total intake and output?
 9. What are his dietary restrictions, if any?
 10. How long has he been in the hospital?
 11. Has he had any pain medication? When?
 12. What is his TPR this morning?

YOUR ANSWER

CORRECT ANSWER

Ineffective.

3

Information that will assist the nurse to make decisions about the care of the patient is provided in a number of resources.

When should the nurse consult these resources?

YOUR ANSWER

CORRECT ANSWER

Before she becomes actively involved in caring for the patient, or as soon as possible after she comes on duty.

4

One major source of information about each patient is his kardex card. It contains the following information:

1. General information about the patient.
2. Physician's orders to be carried out by nursing personnel.
3. Observations made by nursing personnel which aid in the care of the patient.

In Appendix A, you will find four kardex cards, each for a different patient. Refer to them as you go on through the next frames.

(Go on to the next frame.)

5

The following general information is recorded in the lower inside portion of the kardex card:

1. Patient's religion and age.
2. When the patient was admitted to the hospital, his location in the hospital, and the service to which he has been assigned, e.g., medicine, allergy.
3. The patient's diagnosis, and what surgical measures, if any, have taken place.
4. Type of diet, and whether intake and output are to be measured.

In the next frame, you will be asked to extract the above information from the two kardexes found on pages 151-152 and 158-159.

(Go on to the next frame.)

6

Write down the general information about Miss Groom and Mr. Willoughby.
(For unfamiliar abbreviations, see the Glossary in Appendix A.)

YOUR ANSWER

CORRECT ANSWER

Miss Groom: age 37
Protestant
Admitted 4 days ago
In bed 5
Urology Service
Diagnosis: Uremia
Diet: 40 Gm. protein
Measure I and O

Mr. Willoughby: age 45
Catholic
Admitted 1 week ago
In bed 14
Thoracic Surgery Service
Diagnosis: Cancer Rt. Lung
Surgery: Rt. Lobectomy 4 days ago
Diet: Soft
Measure I and O

7

The rest of the kardex card provides information about the care of the patient. This includes measurements that the physician wants the nurse to make, treatments to be carried out for the patient, and any limitations on the patient's activity or on amount of fluid intake. Medications, both standing and p.r.n., and any preparation required for scheduled appointments are also included.

Review Mr. Willoughby's and Miss Groom's kardex cards, and answer the following questions:

1. What and how much can each patient have to eat and drink?

YOUR ANSWER

CORRECT ANSWER

| | Miss Groom | | Mr. Willoughby |

1. a. 40 Gm. protein diet.
   b. Restrict fluids to 800 cc./day.
   c. NPO after midnight.

1. a. Soft diet.
   b. Encourage fluids to 3000 cc./day.

2. What kind of activity has been ordered by the doctor?

YOUR ANSWER

CORRECT ANSWER

2. a. SCB

2. a. May not lie on right side.
   b. Chair for 30" t.i.d.

3. What treatments are ordered? How frequently?

YOUR ANSWER

CORRECT ANSWER

3. a. Special skin care b.i.d.
   b. Special mouth care q. 2°.

3. a. Cough and turn q. 2°.
   b. Deep breathe q. 2°.
   c. Range of motion to right arm and shoulder t.i.d.
   d. Chest tubes to bubble suction continuously.

4. What measurements should the nurse take? How frequently?

YOUR ANSWER

CORRECT ANSWER

4.   a. I and O
      b. TPR q. 4°.
      c. VS q. 2°.
      d. Weight q. d.

4.   a. I and O.
      b. TPR q. 4°
      c. VS q.i.d.

5. What standing medications has the doctor ordered? Route? Dosage? Frequency?

YOUR ANSWER

CORRECT ANSWER

5.   a. Librium 10 mgm. (o) t.i.d.

5.   a. Procaine penicillin 400,000 U. (IM) b.i.d.

6. What p.r.n. medications have been ordered? Route? Dosage? Frequency?

YOUR ANSWER

CORRECT ANSWER

6.   a. Compazine 10 mgm. (IM) q. 4-6° p.r.n. nausea.

6.   a. Demerol 75 mgm. (IM) q. 3-4° p.r.n. pain.

8

Read the "Guides to Nursing Management" on all four kardex cards found in Appendix A.
What kinds of information are recorded?

YOUR ANSWER

CORRECT ANSWER

Nurses record information which will be helpful to other nursing personnel caring for this patient.
   1. Patient's preferences.
   2. Means the nurse has found effective for carrying out a treatment.
   3. Patient's understanding of the treatment.

9

You have the following conversation with a sixteen year old boy named Fritz Cooper. One of his treatments is "alcohol rub to back followed by heat lamp to sacral area q.i.d.". Fritz has been complaining of a backache, which he says usually only occurs during and immediately after the heat lamp treatment.

Write down what you would put in the "Guides to Nursing Management" on his kardex, after you have read the following interaction.

Nurse: "Perhaps you aren't in a comfortable position while the lamp is on. I'll rub your back with the alcohol and then see if I can make you comfortable for the heat lamp treatment."

Fritz: "Well – okay...."

Nurse: (Draws curtain around unit. Lowers the head of the bed, assists Fritz to lie on his side, uncovers his back, and begins to rub sacral area with alcohol.)

Fritz: "Good grief! Can't you warm that stuff up?"

Nurse: "Yes – I can." (Holds alcohol a while longer in hand before putting it on his back.) "Is that better?"

Fritz: "Yeah." (Stares dreamily into space.) "The guys are playing Baytown tonight. If we beat them, we might have a chance for the championship."

Nurse: "You must have a good team."

Fritz: "Yeah – well, maybe I'll be out in a couple of weeks, and then I can see the last game."

Nurse: "I'm through rubbing your back now. I think if I put a small pillow under your waist, you'll be more comfortable." (Slides pillow under Fritz's waist. Plumps up pillows under his head and shoulders.)

Fritz: "It feels okay *now*."

Nurse: "All right. You let me know how you feel as the treatment progresses. I'll be back to check on you, while the lamp is on."

After you have checked him and have returned in twenty minutes to turn off the heat lamp, Fritz says that he is comfortable, and his back does not ache.

YOUR ANSWER

CORRECT ANSWER

1. Patient prefers warm alcohol for back rub. (Hold in hands prior to applying.)
2. Patient is more comfortable during heat lamp treatment if a small pillow is placed under his waist.

10

The appointment sheet is another source of information which the nurse uses. Patients frequently have treatments or consultations with other medical personnel in or away from their hospital room. The nurse should know when these appointments have been scheduled, so that she will not plan other nursing activities at the same time, and so that she can have the patient ready for the appointment on time. She should also find out if any preparation is required. A list of appointments is kept on the Appointment Schedule which is found on page 150. Look at it now.

(Go on to the next frame.)

11

What appointments are scheduled for Miss Groom and Mr. Willoughby? When? What special preparations are necessary, if any?

YOUR ANSWER

CORRECT ANSWER

Miss Groom has an appointment for kidney function studies at 11:00 A.M. NPO after midnight.

Mr. Willoughby has an appointment for a portable chest x-ray at 9:30 A.M.

12

At the end of each shift, the nurse who has been responsible for the care of certain patients gives a verbal report to the nurse coming on duty, who will be caring for these same patients. This report is a summary of important indicators of the patient's condition (see page 178). The nurse receiving the report should have either the kardex or the information from the kardex written on a worksheet in front of her, so that if any important information is missing, such as an observation or results of a treatment, she can ask the nurse who is giving the report about it.

(Go on to the next frame.)

13

Here is an example of the night nurse reporting to the day nurse at 8:00 A.M. Read through it, and answer the questions below.

Mr. Willoughby was awakened every two hours to cough last night, although he slept in between. He coughed up a moderate amount of thick, whitish-green mucus. He had pain in his right shoulder last evening, and he was given Demerol 75 mgm. (IM) at 7:30 P.M. He hasn't asked for pain medication since then. He moves his arm well through range of motion. The dressing on his incision remains dry, and he's had no drainage through his chest tubes since last evening. So, from 8:00 A.M. yesterday until 8:00 A.M. today, he's had a total of 50 cc. of drainage, which was light red in color. His vital signs of last night at 10:00 P.M. were 130/76, P. 74, and R. 30. TPR this morning is 101^4, 86, and 30. That's down from what it was last night, when it was 102. His oral intake from 8:00 A.M. yesterday through 8:00 A.M. today was 3460 cc.; his output was 1875 cc. He is to have a portable chest x-ray at 9:30 A.M. today.

1. What appointments have been ordered during the oncoming shift? For what time? Has the preparation been carried out up until now?

YOUR ANSWER

CORRECT ANSWER

1. Portable chest x-ray at 9:30 A.M. No special preparation necessary.

2. What are the results of ordered treatments? What are the findings of physician's ordered observations and measurements?

YOUR ANSWER

CORRECT ANSWER

    2. a. Coughed up moderate amount of thick, whitish-green mucus.
        b. Has had total of 50 cc. of light red drainage through chest tube from 8:00 A.M. yesterday through 8:00 A.M. today. No drainage through the night.
        c. Vital signs at 10:00 P.M. last night were 130/76, P. 74, and R. 30.
        d. TPR at 8:00 A.M. today is 101^4, 86, and 30.
        e. Intake=3460 cc. Output=1875 cc.
        f. Moves arm well through range of motion.

    3. What additional observations has the nurse made of the patient's condition? What action was taken? What effect did it have?

YOUR ANSWER

CORRECT ANSWER

    3. Additional observations:
        a. Had pain in right shoulder last night; received Demerol 75 mgm. (IM) apparently with some relief. Has not asked for pain medication since then.
        b. Dressing on incision remains dry.
        c. Slept, except for being awakened to cough.

14

    In the report, the nurse presents three kinds of information about the patient.

    1. Scheduled appointments during the oncoming shift. Preparation required for the appointments and status of the preparations.

    2. Results of ordered treatments. Findings of the physician's ordered observations and measurements.

    3. Additional observations made by the nurse. Action taken and effects of the action.

(Go on to the next frame.)

15

Here is another example of the night nurse reporting to the day nurse at 8:00 A.M. Read through it carefully. Are there any questions about missing information that you, as the day nurse, would ask the night nurse? (Consult Miss Groom's kardex card.)

Miss Groom was nauseated last evening. She had Compazine at 6:30 P.M. and has been okay since then. She was quite tired and fell asleep at 8:30 P.M., but slept fitfully all night. She woke up frequently, and, at one time, around 3:00 A.M. sat right up in bed and said, "Is dinner ready?" She didn't know where she was, but then she calmed down and went to sleep. When she woke up again around 4:30 A.M., she was oriented. Her skin is very dry, so I put some more lotion on it. Her vital signs are stable at 156/110, P. 86, and R. 28. She's been NPO since midnight for a kidney function test this morning at 11:00 A.M. She weighs 131 pounds this morning; she's gained a pound since yesterday.

YOUR ANSWER

CORRECT ANSWER

    a. What is her most recent temperature?

    b. Has she had mouth care? Condition of her mouth.

    c. What is her total intake and output?

16

At the beginning of this program, you considered the problems of the nurse who tried to care for Mr. Holmes without information. In the preceding pages, we have shown you where the nurse can gather the information that answers the questions about Mr. Holmes' care. Here are the questions again. Consult any resources you wish, and answer each of the questions. The nurse is caring for the patient from 8:00 A.M. until noon.

    1. What is his diagnosis?

YOUR ANSWER

CORRECT ANSWER

    1. Rheumatoid arthritis.

    2. What treatments are scheduled?

YOUR ANSWER

CORRECT ANSWER

    2. Heating pad to right shoulder, range of motion to all extremities.

    3. How many times a day should each treatment be done and, where appropriate, for how long?

YOUR ANSWER

CORRECT ANSWER

    3. Heating pad for 30 '' q.i.d., range of motion b.i.d.

    4. How does he like them done?

YOUR ANSWER

CORRECT ANSWER

    4. Likes to do range of motion after breakfast and after supper, when he is less tired. Needs help with lower extremities.

    5. What appointments are scheduled? At what time? What preparation is necessary?

YOUR ANSWER

CORRECT ANSWER

    5. P.T. appointment at 8:30 A.M. Early breakfast.

    6. What are his activity limitations and specifically prescribed activities?

YOUR ANSWER

CORRECT ANSWER

    6. He can get out of bed, and he must ambulate t.i.d.

    7. What medications are ordered? At what time?

YOUR ANSWER

CORRECT ANSWER

    7. Buffered aspirin, Prednisone, Diuril, and E.C. KCl at 10:00 A.M.

    8. Is it necessary to measure intake and output? What was yesterday's total intake and output?

YOUR ANSWER

CORRECT ANSWER

    8. Yes, must measure I and O. Yesterday's totals: I=2350 cc., O=1700 cc.

    9. What are his dietary restrictions, if any?

YOUR ANSWER

CORRECT ANSWER

    9. No added salt diet.

    10. How long has he been in this hospital?

YOUR ANSWER

CORRECT ANSWER

    10. He's been in the hospital for one week.

    11. Has he had any pain medication? When?

YOUR ANSWER

CORRECT ANSWER

    11. Had Darvon 65 mgm. for pain in his right shoulder last evening at 9:30 P.M.

    12. What is his TPR this morning?

YOUR ANSWER

CORRECT ANSWER

    12. His TPR at 8:00 A.M. is 99^6, 74, and 26.

17

    We have just shown that there are records such as the kardex, the appointment sheet, and the verbal report at the end of each shift by which nurses communicate about patients for whom they are caring. Each patient also has a chart (see Appendix A), which includes the patient's history, laboratory records, and nursing notes, which the nurse uses to inform the physician and other qualified personnel about the patient's condition. The pages that the nurse fills out are in the front of the chart.

(Go on to the next frame.)

18

    Look at the sample chart of Mr. Willoughby as you read this frame.

    Since the physician is normally with the patient for only a few minutes once or twice a day, he must rely on others to keep him informed on the patient's condition. The nurse records observations and any of the patient's treatments or activities as follows:

    1. Temperature, pulse, respiration, and blood pressure (on the graphic sheets).

    2. Intake and output (on intake and output record).

3. Medications and times they were given (on medication record).

4. Treatments given and patient's response, as well as other observations of the patient's condition (on nursing notes).

(Go on to the next frame.)

19

Since the nurse, unlike the doctor, is continually with the patient, it is her responsibility to be aware of the patient's condition. Her observations suggest ways in which the patient's care should be modified, either as directed by the physician or as initiated by the nurse. The next frames are designed to teach you how to find out about the patient's condition.

(Go on to the next frame.)

20

The nurse gets clues from the patient's chart, his kardex, and the verbal report that suggest observations she should make.

(Go on to the next frame.)

21

Listed below are examples of treatments from the kardex and two types of observations the nurse is expected to make. What are the two types of observations the nurse has made using the kardex information?

Nurse Observation

Kardex	*Type One*	*Type Two*
1. Intravenous therapy 1000 cc. 5% D/W.	1. Check amount of fluid in the IV bottle, rate of flow of fluid, whether fluid is flowing into vein.	1. Check IV insertion site on arm for edema and erythema.
2. Appendectomy two days ago.	2. None.	2. Check dressing to note if there is any drainage, and, if so, what the drainage looks like.
3. Alternating pressure mattress.	3. See if the pressure ridges of the mattress are alternately inflating and deflating.	3. None.
4. Cast on left leg from toes to knee.	4. None.	4. See if there are any pressure areas under the edges of the cast. Also, see if circulation is adequate to toes. Note any drainage on, or odor from, the cast.
5. Foley catheter to dependent drainage.	5. See if tubing connecting the catheter with the drainage bag is patent.	5. Note color and amount of urine.

YOUR ANSWER

CORRECT ANSWER

1. Observations of the functioning of the equipment.

2. Observations of the patient associated with the treatment.

22

At first, when you are a nursing student, you will probably not know how to operate all of the equipment and make all of the observations connected with it. You will learn about this throughout your nursing education. When you do not understand how equipment works or what observations to make regarding it, you should ask your instructor or another nurse.

(Go on to the next frame.)

23

We have extracted from the kardex card and the nursing report one bit of information for each of four patients. Read the information, and write down what observations you would make on the basis of this information.

1. "Mr. Smith's wound has a moderate amount of sero-sanguinous drainage."

YOUR ANSWER

CORRECT ANSWER

1. Check to see the amount of drainage on the dressing when you first see the patient.

2. Mrs. Roberts: oxygen tent.

YOUR ANSWER

CORRECT ANSWER

2. Check the gauges to see that the flow rate of oxygen is correct.

3. Mr. Thomas: Russell's traction to fractured right leg. (This is a system of ropes, weights, and pulleys which maintain the leg in balance to promote healing.)

YOUR ANSWER

CORRECT ANSWER

3. Check to see that the weights do not touch the floor, and that the ropes move unhindered.

4. "Mrs. James' right wrist is edematous (swollen) due to her intravenous therapy infiltrating into the subcutaneous tissue last night. It looks about twice the size of her left wrist."

YOUR ANSWER

CORRECT ANSWER

4. Observe the amount of edema in Mrs. James' wrist.

(If you did not know what observations to make and said that you would ask your instructor, this is correct under these circumstances.)

24

The nurse could make all of the preceding observations without asking the patient any questions. For example, observation alone was sufficient to determine whether there was drainage on the dressing, whether the fluid from the IV bottle was flowing into the vein, and whether the IV site was erythematous (red) or edematous (swollen).

There are times when direct observation alone is not enough. The nurse gets clues from various resources including the patient, but she must combine these clues with questions to the patient. For example:

1. She notices that an IV site is erythematous and edematous. This suggests that it is painful, but she needs to ask the patient if it is, in fact, painful.

2. She has learned from verbal report that the patient did not sleep well. She needs to ask him if he is tired.

3. She walks into the patient's room. He is yawning and his eyes are half closed. This may indicate that he is sleepy, but she needs to ask the patient to be sure.

(Go on to the next frame.)

25

In the examples below are parts of the verbal report and observations the nurse has just made about the patient's condition. Read each item and then write down a question you might ask the patient in order to complete your information about the patient.

1. The verbal report states, "The patient was nauseated during the night."

YOUR ANSWER

CORRECT ANSWER

1. "Are you still nauseated this morning?"
   "Have you been able to eat anything this morning?"

2. You see that the patient is curled up in his bed under a light blanket.

YOUR ANSWER

CORRECT ANSWER

2. "Are you chilly?"

3. The verbal report states, "The patient had a lot of pain in his right leg last night and took some pain medication just before he went to sleep. It apparently relieved his pain."

YOUR ANSWER

CORRECT ANSWER

3. "Have you had any more pain in your right leg since last night?"

4. The patient has an elastic bandage wrapped around his wrist. You notice that he is rubbing his hand and flexing his fingers.

YOUR ANSWER

CORRECT ANSWER

4. "Does your hand feel numb?"
   "Does your hand feel prickly?"

26

Much of nursing care involves processing information from the patient and from a variety of resources, and then acting upon it. We have shown you that the nurse needs to have a base line of information about her patient as she begins to care for him. She gets this information by direct observation of the patient and his equipment and by questioning the patient. For example, the kardex lists ordered treatments. The nurse knows that she should check the functioning of any equipment involved and determine the effectiveness of the treatment to date. Similarly, resource information and the nurse's observations of the patient allow her to pose questions specifically related to that patient. This is better than asking the patient, "How do you feel?", because it allows the nurse to get more specific information about the patient's condition faster.

(Go on to the next frame.)

27

Here is the night report again for Mr. Willoughby. His kardex card is found on pages 158 and 159. Look at both the report ant his kardex card.

Write down three items of information that you would like to get initially. For each one state what you would do to get this information.

"Mr. Willoughby was awakened every two hours to cough last night, although he slept in between. He coughed up a moderate amount of thick, whitish-green mucus. He had pain in his right shoulder last evening, and he was given Demerol 75 mgm. (IM) at 7:30 P.M. He hasn't asked for pain medication since then. He moves his arm well through range of motion. The dressing on his incision remains dry, and he's had no drainage through his chest tubes since last evening. So, from 8:00 A.M. yesterday until 8:00 A.M. today, he's had a total of 50 cc. of drainage, which was light red in color. His vital signs last night at 10:00 P.M. were 130/76, P. 74, and R. 30. TPR this morning is 101^4, 86, and 30. That's down from what it was last night, when it was 102. His oral intake from 8:00 A.M. yesterday through 8:00 A.M. today was 3460 cc.; his output was 1875 cc. He is to have a portable chest x-ray at 9:30 A.M. today."

(The nurse can accept the last measurements of TPR, VS, intake, and output as accurate and does not need to include these in her initial observations with Mr. Willoughby.)

YOUR ANSWER

CORRECT ANSWER

Necessary Information	*How Obtained*

Necessary Information

1. Is Mr. Willoughby's right shoulder painful?
2. Extent of drainage on his dressing.
3. Amount and color of drainage through chest tubes.

Correct but not necessary initially

4. Amount and character of any mucus coughed up.
5. Is he tired?
6. How does he do range of motion exercises?

How Obtained

1. Ask him:
   "Have you had any more pain in your right shoulder since last evening?" or "How does your right shoulder feel this morning?"
2. Look at dressing.
3. Look at calibrated bottle on the end of the drainage tubes.
4. "Have you coughed up any mucus this morning?"
5. "How did you sleep last night?"
6. Observe him move his arm through range of motion.

28

At the same time the nurse is observing the patient and asking him questions, she should also be assessing his circulation, breathing, position and movement, mood, and sensory perception. These five categories comprise one method of assessment. The nurse should use some method of assessment with all patients to structure her observations.

(Go on to the next frame.)

29

The five categories are listed below, together with one observation that might be made about the patient. In the blank space, list another observation that the nurse might make for each category.

Category

1. Circulation.

2. Breathing.

3. Position and movement.

4. Mood.

5. Sensory perception

Observation

1. a. Is the patient's skin pale? Flushed?

YOUR ANSWER

b.

CORRECT ANSWER

1. b. Is his skin warm or cold to the touch?

2. a. Is the patient having difficulty breathing? Is his breathing irregular?

YOUR ANSWER

b.

CORRECT ANSWER

2. b. Is he coughing?

3. a. Are there any parts of the patient's body that he has difficulty moving?

YOUR ANSWER

b.

CORRECT ANSWER

3. b. Is the patient slouched?

4. a. Is the patient wringing his hands? Talking constantly?

YOUR ANSWER

b.

CORRECT ANSWER

4. b. Is the patient laughing? Crying?

5. a. Can the patient hear?

YOUR ANSWER

b.

CORRECT ANSWER

5. b. Can the patient see? (Or equivalent response.)

30

In the program, we have briefly described one method of assessing the patient. You will be learning to apply this method (or one like it) throughout your nursing studies.

(Go on to the next frame.)

31

When the nurse receives data from the resources (the kardex, the verbal report, and the patient) at the beginning of each shift, she should also know the previous pattern or course of the patient's illness. Listed below are examples of the prior pattern of the patient's illness, 8:00 A.M. data, the nurse's subsequent observations of the patient, and the changes indicated in the patient's condition.

32

Read the examples, and fill in the last column in examples 2a and 2b.

Prior Pattern	*8:00 A.M. Data Verbal Report*	*Subsequent Observation*	*Change in Patient's Condition?*
1. a. Mr. White has been hospitalized for four days to undergo diagnostic tests. He has had no fever.	1. a. Mr. White's TPR is 98, 70, and 24.	1. a. At noon, the nurse discovers that Mr. White's TPR is 103, 84, and 30.	1. a. Yes, marked elevation of TPR over previous readings.
b. Mr. Black has been hospitalized for two days with pneumonia. He has had a continuous fever.	b. Mr. Black's TPR is 102⁴, 86, and 32.	b. At noon, the nurse notes that Mr. Black's TPR is 102, 82, and 30.	b. No marked change in TPR. TPR remains elevated, as it has for the past two days.
	Nurse's Observations		
2. a. Joe Green, age sixteen, was in a driving accident five days ago. Since then, he has lost all feeling in both legs and cannot move them.	2. a. Patient continues to have no feeling in, or movement of, his legs.	2. a. At midmorning, Joe Green states that his legs feel prickly, and he is able to wiggle his toes.	**YOUR ANSWER**
			CORRECT ANSWER
			2. a. Yes, previously unobserved prickly sensation and limited motion suggest a change in Joe Green's condition.
b. Mr. Brown, age sixty-eight, suffered a stroke two months ago that has left him with prickly sensations in his legs. He cannot move them and can only wiggle his toes.	b. Patient continues to have prickly sensations in his legs and has only the ability to move his toes.	b. At midmorning, Mr. Brown continues to have prickly sensations in his legs and has only the ability to wiggle his toes.	**YOUR ANSWER**
			CORRECT ANSWER
			b. No, continued prickly sensation and limited motion indicate no change in Mr. Brown's condition.

33

Why is it important that the nurse should know both the prior pattern of the patient's illness and the recent data concerning his condition?

YOUR ANSWER

CORRECT ANSWER

It enables her to determine if there has been a change in the patient's condition and allows her to make more reliable inferences as to what these changes might mean.

34

The nurse should have sufficient knowledge about disease conditions and the prior pattern of the patient's illness, so that when changes occur in the patient's condition, she can make reliable inferences about what the changes mean.

For example, the marked elevation of Mr. White's temperature might be a clue to his diagnosis. The return of limited motion and sensation in Joe Green's legs may indicate an improvement in his condition.

These changes in Mr. White's and Joe Green's conditions have implications for nursing action.

(Go on to the next frame.)

35

Below are the changes observed in Mr. Black, Mr. White, Joe Green, and Mr. Brown. Turn back to the preceding frames for additional information about them, if you wish. Nursing actions for Joe Green and Mr. Brown are given. Indicate the nursing actions implied for Mr. White and Mr. Black.

Observed Changes

1. a. Previously unobserved prickly sensation and limited motion suggest a change in Joe Green's condition.
   b. Continued prickly sensation and limited motion indicate no change in Mr. Brown's condition.

Actions

1. a. The nurse tells the physician, so that he can assess the change in Joe Green's condition and determine whether the course of treatment should be altered.
   b. Since Mr. Brown's condition has not changed, the nurse continues the treatments already ordered.

YOUR ANSWER

CORRECT ANSWER

2. a. Marked elevation of Mr. White's TPR over previous readings.
   b. No marked change in TPR. Mr. Black's TPR remains elevated, as it has for the past two days.

2. a. The nurse would tell the physician, so that he can use this additional information in making a diagnosis.

YOUR ANSWER

CORRECT ANSWER

   b. Since Mr. Black's condition has not changed, the nurse continues the treatments already ordered.

36

Listed below are observations which the nurse has made of several patients. Fill in an appropriate nursing action.

Observations

Nursing Action

1. Mrs. Brown has an intravenous feeding of 5% dextrose in normal saline, which is to continue for the next two days. Each bottle contains 1000 cc., which runs in over an eight hour period. The amount of fluid remaining in the bottle is only 50 cc.

YOUR ANSWER

CORRECT ANSWER

1. Prepare the next bottle of fluid, and exchange it with the one that is nearly empty.

2. Miss Rix has a cast on her right arm. The nurse notices that her right hand is blue, and her fingers are swollen.

YOUR ANSWER

CORRECT ANSWER

2. Notify the physician that the circulation appears to be impaired.

3. Mr. Johnson has a naso-gastric tube attached to low suction. The physician's order states: irrigate naso-gastric tube with 50 cc. normal saline p.r.n. to keep tubing open. The nurse notices that there is no drainage coming through the naso-gastric tubing, and the patient is complaining of fullness and pain in his abdomen.

YOUR ANSWER

CORRECT ANSWER

3. The nurse irrigates the tubing with 50 cc. of normal saline, in order to try to open the blocked tubing. If she is unable to do so, she notifies the physician.

4. Mr. Richards, who has had a high fever for two days, awakens from a nap and is diaphoretic. His gown and bed clothes are soaked with perspiration.

YOUR ANSWER

CORRECT ANSWER

4. The nurse gets him a clean dry gown, changes all of the bed clothes, and checks his present TPR.

37

In the preceding frame, there may have been some actions which you did not know. The same thing may happen when you are caring for a patient.

What would you do?

YOUR ANSWER

CORRECT ANSWER

You would ask either your instructor or another nurse about what the appropriate action would be.

38

Take out Mr. Willoughby's kardex card and chart, and look at it again. Since Mr. Willoughby had his chest surgery four days ago, he has been progressing satisfactorily. Until yesterday he has had no fever and has coughed up normal-appearing, yellow-white mucus. His incision appears to be healing well. A couple of times, after doing range of motion exercises, his right shoulder has become painful, and he has received pain medication.

Below are listed data that the nurse receives at 8:00 A.M. (either from report or from her own observations) and subsequent observations that the nurse makes of Mr. Willoughby. Look at these in addition to the information you have about the prior course of Mr. Willoughby's recovery from surgery, and then decide what changes the nurse observes and what subsequent actions she should take.

8:00 A.M. Data	Subsequent Observations	Change in Patient's Condition?	Nursing Action
1. Patient states that his right shoulder is not painful.	1. At 11:00 A.M., after doing his range of motion exercises, he complains of pain in his right shoulder.	**YOUR ANSWER**	**YOUR ANSWER**
		CORRECT ANSWER 1. Yes, pain in the patient's right shoulder is a change from 8:00 A.M. Previously, the same thing has happened after doing range of motion exercises.	**CORRECT ANSWER** 1. Prepare and administer pain medication: Demerol 75 mgm. (IM).
2. Patient's TPR is 101^4, 86, and 30.	2. At noon, his TPR is 101, 82, and 28.	**YOUR ANSWER**	**YOUR ANSWER**
		CORRECT ANSWER 2. No, his temperature remains elevated.	**CORRECT ANSWER** 2. Continue with same actions as before.

8:00 A.M. Data	Subsequent Observations	Change in Patient's Condition?	Nursing Action
3. He has been coughing up a moderate amount of greenish-white mucus.	3. At 9:40 A.M., he has a severe coughing spell and expectorates a mucus plug tinged with bright red blood.	**YOUR ANSWER**	**YOUR ANSWER**
		CORRECT ANSWER 3. A marked change from 8:00 A.M.	**CORRECT ANSWER** 3. Notify the physician immediately.
4. Upon questioning, the patient states that he does not feel particularly tired this morning and is looking forward to getting up in the chair.	4. At 10:15 A.M., after being up in the chair for ten minutes, he says that he feels weak and tired.	**YOUR ANSWER**	**YOUR ANSWER**
		CORRECT ANSWER 4. Yes.	**CORRECT ANSWER** 4. Assist him back to bed, and observe him periodically to see if he still feels weak or if he becomes more rested.

Part II

STRUCTURING THE PROFESSIONAL RELATIONSHIP

A. THE PROFESSIONAL INTERACTION

39

In any professional role, there are certain goals to be accomplished. These goals determine the content of the communication that occurs between the professional and his client. Unlike a social conversation, which may cover a wide range of topics and may occur spontaneously, a professional interaction is directed toward meeting the goals of the client.

(Go on to the next frame.)

40

For example, the professional could err by structuring the relationship as though it were a social one. Consider the following unlikely interaction between a lawyer and his client, and state why the lawyer is not effective.

The client, Mr. Katz, enters Mr. Locke's office.

Mr. Katz: "I need to talk to you, because some fool in a station wagon rammed into my sports car last week, and I've had a sore back ever since. He refused to pay any damages, and I want to sue him!"

Mr. Locke: "Do you know who it was that hit you?"

Mr. Katz: "Yes, it's Joe Hicks."

Mr. Locke: "Hmm. . . ." (Locke thoughtful. Then his glance falls on Mr. Katz' college ring.) "Say! Did you go to Catall University?"

Mr. Katz: "Yes."

Mr. Locke: "Same here! Class of '59! When were you there?" (And the conversation dissolves into a reminiscence of college days.)

YOUR ANSWER

CORRECT ANSWER

Because he did not direct the interview to meet the goals of the client.

41

Read the next two interactions between Miss Jenkins and Mrs. Robinson. Which one is more effective and why?

Interaction A

Miss Jenkins: "Good Morning, Mrs. Robinson. How did you sleep last night?"

Mrs. Robinson: "Well, I have a headache, I've had it for quite a while."

Miss. Jenkins: "I get headaches fairly frequently myself. I think it's the damp weather or something. It bothers me whenever I go out."

Mrs. Robinson: "Yes — well, I've had mine for about three hours now."

Miss Jenkins: "Really? Mine usually last longer than that, about five or six hours. Sometimes they go away, and sometimes I have to take something for them."

Mrs. Robinson: "Hmm. . . . do you suppose you might bring me something for my headache?"

Miss Jenkins: "Oh! Oh, yes! I'll go get you a pain pill right away."

Interaction B

Miss Jenkins:	"Good morning, Mrs. Robinson. How did you sleep last night?"
Mrs. Robinson:	"Not very well, I have a headache. I've had it for quite a while."
Miss Jenkins:	"How long have you had it?"
Mrs. Robinson:	"I guess about three hours."
Miss Jenkins:	"What kind of pain do you have?"
Mrs. Robinson:	"Just kind of a dull pain, here, over my temple."
Miss Jenkins:	"Have you had any pain medication for it?"
Mrs. Robinson:	"No, not since last night."
Miss Jenkins:	"Oh, I'll get you some and be right back."

YOUR ANSWER

CORRECT ANSWER

Interaction B was the more effective because she directed the conversation toward the goal of alleviating the patient's headache.

She structured the relationship professionally rather than socially.

BEHAVIORAL OBJECTIVE:

When a patient asks the student a personal question, she answers briefly and redirects the conversation to another topic. (Frames 42–45)

42

The nurse may make every attempt to keep her personal life out of the interaction with the patient, but the patient may attempt to establish the relationship on a personal basis.

When the patient asks the nurse a personal question, there are two things that the nurse should keep in mind. One, she should keep her answer brief, because as a nurse she should not monopolize the conversation and should try to keep it focused primarily on the patient. Two, she has the right as an individual to decide what, if any, personal information she will give to another individual.

(Go on to the next frame.)

43

Read the following two examples. In the first example, Miss Johnson focused on herself rather than on the patient. Compare what she did in the second example with what she did in the first.

1. How does she answer Mrs. Baxter's question?
2. What does she do to encourage Mrs. Baxter to pursue a new topic?

Example I

Miss Johnson:	"Here is your bath water, Mrs. Baxter."
Mrs. Baxter:	"Thank you. I think you are going to be a fine nurse. How did you happen to decide to go into nursing?"

Miss Johnson:	"I liked the health sciences and nursing gives you more real contact with people than the others. You can really see results, like after you've rubbed someone's back or made them more comfortable in some way. It's so nice to be appreciated."
Mrs. Baxter:	"That's very interesting."

Example II

Miss Johnson:	"Here is your bath water, Mrs. Baxter."
Mrs. Baxter:	"Thank you. I think you are going to be a fine nurse. How did you happen to decide to go into nursing?"
Miss Johnson:	"I liked the health sciences and thought nursing was a good choice for a woman. Would you like to wash your face and arms? I'll be back in a minute and help you with the rest."
Mrs. Baxter:	"Fine. I'll ring when I'm ready."

YOUR ANSWER

CORRECT ANSWER

1. Miss Johnson answered the question briefly.
2. She returned the focus of the discussion to Mrs. Baxter.

44

Generally, the conversation can be directed away from the nurse without actually cutting the patient off, i.e., by giving a minimal answer and redirecting the focus of the conversation to the patient. However, sometimes the patient persists in asking personal questions, as she does in the example below. Read this example and then state how Miss Zander finally handled this.

Miss Zander:	"Good morning, Mrs. Baxter. I'm Miss Zander, and I'll be caring for you this morning until noon."
Mrs. Baxter:	"Good morning, Miss Zander. Hmm, Zander — that's kind of an unusual name. Are you from Bay View?"
Miss Zander:	"Yes, I am. How are you this morning, Mrs. Baxter?"
Mrs. Baxter:	(Hurriedly.) "Oh, I'm fine. Is your father the mayor of Bay View?"
Miss Zander:	"Yes, he is. You said you were fine. Did you sleep well last night?"
Mrs. Baxter:	"Yes, very well, thank you. He was really quite a good mayor. I voted for him several times."
Miss Zander:	"If I had been old enough I would have voted for him, too! Now I need to talk with you about planning your care. You have some exercises to do this morning, and I notice that you also have an appointment at 10:00 A.M. Would you like to have your bath now, before your appointment, or later?"
Mrs. Baxter:	"Now would be fine."
Miss Zander:	"Okay, I'll be right back with your bath water."

YOUR ANSWER

CORRECT ANSWER

Miss Zander explicitly stated what goal had to be accomplished.

45

You are assigned to care for Mrs. Fulton. If you wish, look at her data again to refresh your memory.

It's now 11:20 A.M. Mrs. Fulton has finished doing the postural drainage, and you have helped her back to bed. The head of her bed is elevated, and she looks thoughtfully out of the window. She turns to look at you and says, "Thank you so much for helping me this morning. You seem to enjoy helping other people. Do you like nursing?"

What would you say to Mrs. Fulton?

YOUR ANSWER

CORRECT ANSWER

"Yes, I do enjoy helping others. Since this is such a large part of nursing, I think I'm going to like it very much. You look a little more rested now than you did earlier this morning."

(Or equivalent response in which you answered briefly and redirected the topic of conversation.)

BEHAVIORAL OBJECTIVE:

When a patient asks for confidential information about another patient, the student informs him that the information is confidential. She also assures him that she can understand his interest and redirects the conversation to another topic. (Frames 46–57)

46

There is one situation in which professional ethics require that communication about certain topics be discouraged. This situation is analogous to that of the physician, minister, and lawyer whose communications with their clients are privileged. *The Code for Professional Nurses* adopted by the American Nurse's Association states that "the nurse respects and holds in confidence all information of a confidential nature obtained in the course of nursing work unless required by law to divulge it." This means that, except when she is talking with other members of the health team who are responsible for the health care of the patient, she does not reveal the patient's diagnosis, his prognosis, or details about his personal life.

(Go on to the next frame.)

47

Here are examples of questions that patients or others may ask the nurse that she is not ethically permitted to answer.

Diagnosis:

    1. "What's wrong with Mr. Glass? He seems very sick."

    2. "It's too bad about Miss Rogers having leukemia, isn't it?"

    3. "I know that Mr. Sebastian was having blood tests yesterday. What were the results?"

Prognosis:

    1. "Johnnie Wills has been here for two months, and he seems to be getting sicker and sicker. Do you think he'll ever get out alive?"

    2. "Mrs. Anthony told me that she has Hodgkin's disease. Do people ever get well from that?"

    3. "I know that Mr. MacPhee got his hand crushed in an automobile accidnt. Will he ever be able to play the piano again?"

Details of Personal Life:

    1. "That young girl is walking around here so depressed. What's she got to be depressed about?"

    2. "Mr. Tiffin's wife hasn't been here to visit him for five days. Aren't they getting along?"

3. "Poor Mrs. Tupper! She's been here for two weeks already! How can they ever afford to pay her medical bills with her husband out of work and six children at home?"

(Go on to the next frame.)

48

In situations like those in the preceding frame, the nurse wants to convey to the patient that she and other members of the health team are prohibited by professional ethics from revealing to one patient what is considered privileged information about another.

If she is successful, the following goals will be met:

1. The patient will not interpret her refusal to answer as having dire implications.
2. The patient will be less likely to feel uncomfortable about having asked the question.
3. The patient will be less likely to continue to try to find out about another patient's condition.

(Go on to the next frame.)

49

Suppose that the patient asks the nurse, "Does Mr. Smith have leukemia?" Listed below are five responses that the nurse might make to the question together with interpretations that the patient might make of her response. Which response is best in terms of the goals listed in the preceding frame?

Nurse Response:	*Possible Interpretations:*
1. "Really, Mr. Brown, that should be no concern of yours."	1. a. "Apparently, I shouldn't have asked the question, because she is irritated that I did."
	b. "He must have leukemia, or she would have said that he didn't."
2. "I don't know. The test results aren't back yet."	2. a. "There is a good chance that he has leukemia, or they wouldn't be doing the tests."
	b. "She didn't refuse to answer my question; she just didn't know. So, I'll ask again later."
3. "No one on the staff is permitted to talk about one patient's condition to another patient."	3. a. "I guess I shouldn't have asked the question, but I'm really worried about him, and she didn't seem to understand that."
4. "I don't know."	4. a. "She isn't very well informed. I'll ask someone else later."
	b. "She is just evading the question. I'll bet he does have leukemia."
5. "I can understand that you're interested in Mr. Smith, but no one on the staff is permitted to talk about one patient's condition to another patient."	5. a. "I guess she can't answer it, even though she does recognize that I'm concerned about him."

YOUR ANSWER

CORRECT ANSWER

Response number five is best.

50

In a written program we cannot convey how facial expression, tone of voice, rate of speaking, and attentiveness affect the meaning of the same spoken words. The manner in which the nurse speaks must be consistent with the words she speaks in order to convey the desired meaning. Below we have tried to show what different interpretations could occur depending upon the manner in which the nurse makes the reply — "I can understand that you're interested in Mr. Smith, but no one on the staff is permitted to talk about one patient's condition with another patient." (Say the sentences to yourself as directed in the column on the left.)

1. Say slowly and quietly with frequent pauses and evade looking at the patient directly.

2. Say abruptly, with emphasis on the words "no one" and the last "patient," while staring fixedly at the patient.

3. Say at usual speed, without special emphasis, while looking attentively at the patient.

1. "He probably has leukemia."

2. "She thought I should have known better than to ask *that!*"

3. "I guess she can't answer it, even though she does recognize that I'm concerned about him."

(Go on to the next frame.)

51

You have been caring for Mr. Craig and Mr. Johnson for two weeks. Mr. Johnson has amyotrophic lateral sclerosis, from which it is highly unlikely he will recover. Mr. Craig says to you, "Mr. Johnson has been here for two weeks, and he's getting weaker and weaker. I wonder if he will leave the hospital alive? Is he going to die?"

What do you say to Mr. Craig?

YOUR ANSWER

CORRECT ANSWER

"Mr. Craig, I know you are interested in Mr. Johnson, but no one on the staff is permitted to talk about one patient's condition to another patient." (Or equivalent response.)

52

If a patient asks a question about another patient who has died, ethically the nurse may tell the patient that the other patient has died and when he died. However, she should not answer any other questions which might then be raised about the patient's death or about his disease condition prior to death.

(Go on to the next frame.)

53

Below are two examples of the nurse responding to the patient's question, "What's the matter with Mrs. Trueblood? She seems to be so sick." *Example II* is more effective. Why?

Example I

"I'm sorry, Mrs. Baker, but no one on the staff is permitted to talk about one patient's condition to another patient."

Example II

"I'm sorry, Mrs. Baker, but no one on the staff is permitted to talk about one patient's condition to another patient. You said a minute ago that you had difficulty sleeping last night?"

YOUR ANSWER

CORRECT ANSWER

Example II is more effective, because the nurse has asked the patient to respond to a question on another topic.

54

Frequently, after the nurse responds and the patient realizes that she cannot answer his question, the patient will begin to talk about something else. However, the nurse makes it more likely that this will happen by suggesting another topic.

(Go on to the next frame.)

55

Information that the nurse already has about the patient provides a direction in which to refocus the topic of conversation. Below we have listed the nurse's source of information and the specific information that the nurse derived from that source. Suppose that the patient, Mr. Carrigan, asks, "What's the matter with Mr. Lucas?" Now, suppose that the nurse replies, "Well, I can appreciate that you're interested in Mr. Lucas, Mr. Carrigan, but information about patients is confidential, and we can't talk about one patient to another." Based on the information in each example, write down four possible things that the nurse could say next.

Source of Information	*Specific Information*
1. Morning report.	1. Mr. Carrigan was awake until 4:00 A.M.
2. Kardex card.	2. Encourage ambulation t.i.d.
3. Previous conversation.	3. He has said that his son will be graduating from college soon.
4. Environmental clues.	4. He has been watching the World Series game on TV.

Possible Verbal Response

YOUR ANSWER

1.

CORRECT ANSWER

1. "I understand you didn't sleep well last night. Are you tired today?"

YOUR ANSWER

2.

CORRECT ANSWER

2. "How have you felt when you're up and walking around?" or "Would you like to walk now or in an hour or so?"

YOUR ANSWER

3.

CORRECT ANSWER

3. "What is your son going to do after he graduates?"

YOUR ANSWER

4.

CORRECT ANSWER

4. "Are you interested in baseball?" or "Who's winning?"

(Obviously, answers will vary somewhat for different students. All correct answers redirect the conversation.)

56

The following interactions both show correct responses by the nurse to questions asked by the patient. How does the nurse's response differ in each example, and why is it correct that her response differ in each example?

Example I

Mr. George: "What's the matter with that man who limps down the hall?"

Miss Rix: "He's another patient here in the hospital. Even though I can understand that you are interested in him, I can't talk about one patient's condition with another patient. How have you been doing with your arm exercises?"

Example II

Mr. George: "You're limping today! What happened to you?"

Miss Rix: (Small laugh) "I tripped on the living room rug and pulled a muscle in my leg. (Pause) How have you been doing with your arm exercises?"

YOUR ANSWER

CORRECT ANSWER

In *Example II*, the nurse gives a brief answer, then refocuses the topic of conversation. In *Example I,* she tells him why she cannot answer the question and refocuses the topic of conversation without giving him any information. Professional ethics do not permit the nurse to supply any information about another patient. However, professional ethics do not prohibit her giving any information about herself.

57

You have been assigned to care for Mr. Holmes this morning. It is now 10:30 A.M. Mr. Holmes has done the range of motion exercises and has applied the heating pad to his right shoulder. You are standing near the bed while Mr. Holmes pulls himself up into a more comfortable position. You have noticed throughout the morning that Mr. Holmes frequently glances at an empty bed part way down the ward and then looks away. This empty bed belongs to Mr. Blackburn. You remember hearing in the morning report that Mr. Blackburn is an eighty-three year old man who developed a high fever and pneumonia last night. With the high fever he became delirious and yelled very loudly, so that he was moved to a bed in the hall. His temperature this morning is still 104°, but he has quieted down somewhat. Mr. Holmes looks again at the empty bed and says, "Poor Mr. Blackburn! He really got sick last night. What was the matter?"

What do you say to Mr. Holmes?

YOUR ANSWER

CORRECT ANSWER

"Mr. Holmes, I can see that you are interested in Mr. Blackburn, but no one on the staff is permitted to talk about one patient's condition to another patient. How is your right shoulder feeling this morning?"

(Or equivalent response.)

B. BASIC ORIENTATION

BEHAVIORAL OBJECTIVES:

The student orients the patient by stating the patient's name, her name, the length of time she will care for the patient, her purpose for being with the patient, and by telling him about any scheduled appointments. (Frames 58– 76)

58

The manner in which the nurse presents herself to the patient structures his perception of what her professional role is. The next frames deal with how the nurse presents herself to the patient.

(Go on to the next frame.)

59

While walking across the campus one day, Ann Jacobs meets Dr. Fox, whom she has as a professor in English 210. She greets him, saying "Good morning, Dr. Fox." How would she feel if he made each of the following replies?
A: "Hello there."
B: "Hello there, Ann."

YOUR ANSWER

CORRECT ANSWER

In B she would know that he knew her name. There might be a stronger feeling of being recognized as an individual.

60

Mr. Gerald Lenski has been a patient in the hospital for two days. He has been in contact with many different people. They have greeted him as follows:

Paperboy: "You want a newspaper? It's ten cents."
Cleaning woman: "Do you want these magazines on the floor?"
Nurse: "Good morning!"
Nurse's aide: "Are you the gall bladder? We need to get a urine specimen."
Nurse 2:   "Mr. Mans — oh, no! You're not he!"

Mr. Lenski lies glumly in bed and thinks, "This hospital is pretty impersonal."

You are a nurse, and you are going in to care for Mr. Lenski today. What is the first thing you would say to him and why?

YOUR ANSWER

CORRECT ANSWER

"Good morning, Mr. Lenski." This shows him that you know who he is and recognize him as an individual.

61

In what way would you expect that his view of you will differ from that of the other people with whom he has been in contact?

YOUR ANSWER

CORRECT ANSWER

He might begin to see you as a person who recognizes him as an individual.

62

If you want to be recognized as an individual, you would say, "Good morning, Mr. Lenski

_____."

YOUR ANSWER

CORRECT ANSWER

My name is Miss Adams or Jane Adams.

63

You call the bank to see if your paycheck has been deposited. You spend fifteen mintues talking with various people until finally the woman who handles your account answers:

Woman: "May I help you?"
You: "Yes, I am Gloria Teedwell. Account # 609-541. Can you tell me if a check for $400.00 has been deposited to my account in the last week?"
Woman: "I will check for you. Please call me back in fifteen minutes."
You: "Thank you." (Click.)

What problem do you have when you try to return the call?

YOUR ANSWER

CORRECT ANSWER

You do not know her name and will have to go through the whole procedure again.

64

Consider two possible situations involving Mr. Carter and a nurse. In both situations there are four other nurses on duty. After you have read the situations, state what action Miss Jacobs would take in each case.

Situation I

Mr. Carter, who had an appendectomy two days ago, requested a pain pill from a nurse he had not seen before. After half an hour, she had still not returned with his pain pill. He put on the light and another nurse, Miss Jacobs, came in. The following interaction took place.

Miss Jacobs: "May I help you, Mr. Carter?"
Mr. Carter: "Yes, Miss Jacobs. I told some nurse I wanted a pain pill half an hour ago, and she said she'd bring it right away, but she hasn't brought it yet."
Miss Jacobs: "What was her name?"
Mr. Carter: "She didn't say, and I don't remember what she looked like."
Miss Jacobs: "I can't bring you the pain pill myself. I'll have to check and see who the nurse was."

YOUR ANSWER

CORRECT ANSWER

I.   Check with all four nurses to find out who saw Mr. Carter.

Situation II

Suppose instead that when Miss Jacobs arrived, Mr. Carter said, "Miss Blackman went to get me a pain pill half an hour ago, and she hasn't brought it yet."

YOUR ANSWER

CORRECT ANSWER

II.   She will go directly to Miss Blackman and find out the cause of the delay.

65

In what way was Miss Jacobs' action expedited by knowing that Miss Blackman was the person responsible?

YOUR ANSWER

CORRECT ANSWER

It allowed Miss Jacobs to communicate immediately with Miss Blackman.

66

When a person in a professional or business role introduces himself to another person by name, it makes it more likely that the other person will recognize him as an individual, and it expedites any future communication with this individual.

(Go on to the next frame.)

67

The Joneses are planning a cocktail and barbecue party Saturday afternoon at 5:00 P.M. in their back yard. Mary and Bill Jones invite their friends in various ways. In the column on the left are the invitations. In the column on the right are their friends' reactions.

1. Bill Jones invites his friend Mack over for a "few drinks Saturday afternoon."

1. Mack and his wife wonder, "What time should we go? What do we wear? Will we eat dinner there? For how long do we need a baby sitter?"

2. The Barretts are invited for cocktails at 5:00 P.M. on Saturday.

2. The Barretts wonder, "Is it for dinner? For how long do we need a baby sitter? What do we wear?"

3. The Charleses are invited for cocktails and dinner at 5:00 P.M.

3. The Charleses wonder, "What do we wear? For how long do we need a baby sitter?"

4. The Dickersons are invited to a cocktail and barbecue party from 5:00 P.M. to 9:00 P.M. on Saturday. Mary Jones reminds them to wear slacks and a sweater, since it will be outside.

4. The Dickersons have all the information they need to plan for the party.

(Go on to the next frame.)

68

In the preceding frame, having more information about the cocktail party and barbecue gave the guests the opportunity to develop more accurate expectations about the party and to make more appropriate plans. Similarly, it is important for the patient to have information. Much of the responsibility for providing this information falls to the nurse. In the next section of the program, we will discuss what the nurse tells the patient when she first sees him.

(Go on to the next frame.)

69

Two nurses come into Mr. Carol's room early Thursday morning.

Miss Johnson: "Good morning, Mr. Carol. I am Miss Johnson, I will be taking care of you today until four o'clock."

Miss Gordon: "Hello, Mr. Carol. I am Miss Gordon. I have brought you some medicine. Here's some water."

Suppose Mr. Carol wants a back rub. Whom would he ask and why?

YOUR ANSWER

CORRECT ANSWER

He would ask Miss Johnson, because she has told him that she was generally responsible for his care that day, while Miss Gordon has stated her specific function.

70

All nurses define for the patient the area of their functioning. The nurse who is responsible for his general care should tell this to the patient so that he will know to whom to direct requests. She should also tell him when her responsibilities will end.

Give an example of how the nurse would convey this last information to the patient.

YOUR ANSWER

CORRECT ANSWER

"I'll be leaving at noon," or "I'll be caring for you until four o'clock," etc.

71

The following incidents occurred in General Hospital last week concerning appointments which were scheduled and noted in patient records.

How might the nurse have prevented the frustrating experiences for the patient and the inconveniences to the staff?

1. The occupational therapist arrives at 11:30 A.M. to help the patient with his project and finds the patient is out of the room.

2. The dietician comes to talk with the patient about his low salt diet at 10:00 A.M. and finds the patient in the middle of his bath. The patient is surprised and upset, because he's been waiting to talk with her since yesterday.

3. The messenger comes at 8:30 A.M. to take the patient for an appointment in the out-patient clinic, just as the patient pours his second cup of coffee. The patient looks disappointed and stomps out of the room after the messenger.

YOUR ANSWER

CORRECT ANSWER

The nurse should have told the patient about the appointments far enough in advance, so that he could have been ready for them.

72

Mrs. Lewis has been in the hospital for two months recovering from a fractured right hip. She usually exercises her right leg by herself for forty-five minutes every day at about 9:30 A.M. However, this particular morning she is to have an x-ray of her hip at 10:00 A.M.

Miss Harlan, the nurse, comes in to see Mrs. Lewis early in the morning. She says, "Hello, Mrs. Lewis. I'm Miss Harlan, and I'll be caring for you today until four o'clock. I see you have a big breakfast there!"

What else does she need to tell the patient soon? And why?

YOUR ANSWER

CORRECT ANSWER

"Mrs. Lewis, you have an appointment for an x-ray at ten o'clock this morning." This gives Mrs. Lewis an opportunity to plan her morning activities. (In this instance, she will have to change the time of her exercises.)

73

All of the units of information that the nurse gives to the patient she is caring for are listed below. Please state the purpose that each serves.

1. "Hello, Mr. Grant."

YOUR ANSWER

CORRECT ANSWER

1. Recognizes the individuality of the patient.

2. "I am Miss James."

YOUR ANSWER

CORRECT ANSWER

2. Recognizes the nurse as an individual and permits communication with person responsible for patient's care.

3. "I will be caring for you today."

YOUR ANSWER

CORRECT ANSWER

3. Defines her nursing responsibilities for the patient.

4. "I will be here until four o'clock."

YOUR ANSWER

CORRECT ANSWER

4. Tells patient how long she is responsible for his care.

5. "You have an appointment at 10:30 A.M. for an x-ray."

YOUR ANSWER

CORRECT ANSWER

5. Allows patient to plan his activities, so that he will be ready for the appointment.

74

These preceding units of information are useful when the nurse orients the patient. Webster defines "orient" as "to acquaint with the existing situation or environment." The five units of information that are included in basic orientation are:

1. Name of patient.
2. Nurse's name.
3. What the nurse will do for the patient.
4. Length of time with the patient.
5. The specific activities or treatments for which the patient is scheduled.

(Go on to the next frame.)

75

Miss Short is caring for Mr. Lang for the first time this morning. She goes in to see him, and the following conversation takes place:

Miss Short: "Good morning, Mr. Lang. I am Miss Short, and I will be caring for you until noon. You have an appointment in physical therapy at 9:30 A.M. I'll help you with your bath before you go."

Mr. Lang: "Whew! That was fast! Uh, could you go over some of that again? I didn't get your name."

What could Miss Short have done that would have made it easier for Mr. Lang to assimilate all the information she was giving him?

YOUR ANSWER

CORRECT ANSWER

She could have paused, deferred some of the information until a few minutes later, or interspersed the orienting information throughout the first few minutes of her conversation.

For example:

Miss Short: "Good morning, Mr. Lang. I am Miss Short."

Mr. Lang: "Oh, good morning, Miss Short."

Miss Short: "I'll be caring for you until noon."

Mr. Lang: "Fine."

Miss Short: "I wanted to tell you that you have an appointment in physical therapy at 9:30 A.M.," etc.

76

You are assigned to care for Mr. Robert Holmes until noon. Look at his data again. At 8:10 A.M. you walk into Mr. Holmes' unit. The shade is half drawn; it is a sunny day, and he is looking out the window. He is sitting in bed, propped up against two pillows, slightly slumped over to one side. His gown is slightly wrinkled; his hair looks unruly. On the bedside stand there are a novel, several get well cards and a food tray with empty dishes. There is a newspaper on the bed beside him. As you approach, he turns his head and begins to smile at you.

How would you orient him? Write your answer in the form of a brief dialogue with the patient, including both your comments and his comments.

YOUR ANSWER

CORRECT ANSWER

Nurse: "Good morning, Mr. Holmes. I am Miss (your name)."
Mr. Holmes: "Good morning, Miss _____."
Nurse: *"I'll be caring for you until noon today."*
Mr. Holmes: "Okay. Well, it certainly is a nice day today."
Nurse: "Yes, it is. Kind of cool, though. I just want to remind you that *you have a physical therapy appointment at 8:30 A.M.* That's in twenty minutes. Is there anything I can help you with, or do for you before you go?
Mr. Holmes: "Yes, I've already had my bath, but I need a clean gown," etc.

Of course, the dialogue will vary, but the five units of information should have been present in the conversation, spacing them to allow the patient to listen and make comments, if he wishes.

You might also have commented on his slumped position, asking if he was comfortable.

C. MODIFIED ORIENTATION

BEHAVIORAL OBJECTIVE:

When a need arises to which she must attend without delay (for example, when the patient is emotionally upset or having difficulty breathing), the student will state minimal orienting information, that is, her name and the patient's name. (Frames 77–85)

77

When the nurse meets the patient for the first time, she presents all the orienting information in the first few minutes of her conversation with him. This gives him the opportunity to develop more accurate expectations about what will be happening to him during the time the nurse is caring for him. However, there are times when it is important that the nurse modify the orienting information by omitting some parts of it. The next section of the program will discuss these modifications.

(Go on to the next frame.)

78

One general rule states that the nurse should omit in the orientation situation that information which the patient already has. For example, her orientation would be different when she meets a patient for the first time from what it would be if she had cared for the same patient for a week. The five parts of orientation are listed on the right. For each situation on the left, list the letters of the parts of orientation on the right that the nurse would state in her initial orientation shortly after 8:00 A.M.

Assume that in each case the nurse has cared for the patient every day for two weeks from 8:00 A.M. to 4:00 P.M.

Situation	*Parts of Orientation*
1. Patient has had an appointment in radiation therapy at 11:00 A.M. every day for two weeks and has another one this morning.	a. Name of patient.
	b. Nurse's name.
YOUR ANSWER	c. What the nurse will do for the patient.
	d. Length of time with the patient.
	e. Telling the patient about specific activities or treatments.

CORRECT ANSWER

1. a.

2. Patient has his first appointment in radiation therapy at 11:00 A.M.

YOUR ANSWER

CORRECT ANSWER

2. a., e.

3. Nurse is leaving at noon today, instead of at 4:00 P.M., when she usually leaves.

YOUR ANSWER

CORRECT ANSWER

3. a., d.

4. Nurse is assigned to passing medications this morning, instead of general patient care.

YOUR ANSWER

CORRECT ANSWER

4. a., c.

79

Even when the nurse is caring for a patient for the first time, she may modify her orientation, depending on the patient's condition. For example, Miss Babcock is assigned to care for Mr. Fosdick for the first time. In report at 8:00 A.M., she learns that the reason for his admission yesterday is a severe pain in the lumbar region of his back. He is receiving pain medication for this: Codeine 64 mgm. and A.S.A. gr. X orally every four hours or as needed for pain. The last time he had the pain medication was 4:00 A.M. As she leaves report at 8:15 A.M., she finds that Mr. Fosdick is repeatedly pressing his call light. She walks into his room and finds him lying stiffly in bed with his hands clenched at his sides. When he sees Miss Babcock, he yells, "My back's been hurting for ten minutes, and nobody's come to help me!"

Which response is better and why?

1. "Good morning, Mr. Fosdick. My name is Miss Babcock, and I will be caring for you today until 4:00 P.M. You have an appointment for an x-ray in forty-five minutes at 9:00 A.M. Tell me about the pain you're having in your back.

2. "I am Miss Babcock, Mr. Fosdick. Tell me about the pain you're having in your back.

YOUR ANSWER

CORRECT ANSWER

The second response is better, because the nurse attends to his most immediate needs first.

80

When a need arises that the nurse must attend to without delay, as in the previous frame, she states only minimal orienting information – her name and the patient's name.

Give two other examples of situations in which the nurse would state only minimal orienting information.

YOUR ANSWER

CORRECT ANSWER

Some examples are:
1. Patient is crying.
2. Patient fell out of bed.
3. Patient is vomiting.
4. Patient is bleeding severely.
5. Patient is having difficulty breathing.
6. Patient is emotionally upset.

81

Even in a situation where there is immediate need, and the patient is in some distress, the nurse states her name and the patient's name. She does this, because it imparts to the patient the feeling that the nurse is somewhat familiar with his case, knows who he is, and is interested in him as an individual. By stating her name, the nurse hopes to make the patient more comfortable with someone he knows, even if it is only by name.

(Go on to the next frame.)

82

Frequently, when the patient has an immediate need that must be met, it is an anxiety-producing situation for him.

Should the nurse have to leave him during this time to get a pain pill or to find someone to help her, the patient's anxiety might be increased.

Therefore, what should the nurse say before leaving?

YOUR ANSWER

CORRECT ANSWER

She should state what she is going to do and when she will be back.

83

After the patient's immediate need has been met, and the situation is more normal, what should the nurse say?

YOUR ANSWER

CORRECT ANSWER

She should tell the patient generally what her functions will be with him, how long she will be with him, and what and when his appointments are.

84

Even when a patient is apparently unconscious, he may be aware of some aspects of his environment. It is quite possible that he may be able to hear or to feel some things that are done to him. Therefore, the nurse tells the patient who she is and briefly describes what she will be doing for him just before she does it, so that, in case the patient can understand her, he will have an idea about what is happening to him.

(Go on to the next frame.)

85

You are assigned to care for Mrs. Nora Fulton for the first time. Look at her data.

It is 8:15 A.M. As you enter the ward, you hear Mrs. Fulton coughing loudly. Dressed in her robe, she is sitting on the edge of the bed with her feet dangling over the side. Her coughing lessens as you approach; however, she continues to take deep breaths. Her face is red, and her eyes are teary. She takes a sip of water from the water pitcher on her bedside stand; it is now empty. Besides the water pitcher and a nearly empty box of tissues, the bedside stand contains nothing. The bed clothes look extremely wrinkled and are pushed back in a heap at the foot of the bed. There are two extra blankets on the bed. You stand quietly at the foot of the bed until Mrs. Fulton catches her breath. Then you say to her: (Quote yourself in one or two sentences.)

YOUR ANSWER

CORRECT ANSWER

"Hello, Mrs. Fulton, I am (your name). That was quite a coughing spell you had. Are you all right?" (Or equivalent response that focuses on her immediate need.)

D. TERMINATION OF CARE

BEHAVIORAL OBJECTIVE:

The student terminates her care of the patient by informing him about a half an hour ahead of time when she will be leaving, by asking if there is anything she can do before she leaves and by placing the call button within reach. (Frames 86–89)

86

Below are two examples of the nurse terminating her care with the patient. Which one is better and why?

Example I

"Mr. Tibbett, I'll be leaving in five minutes. Is there anything I can do for you before I leave?"

Example II

"Mr. Tibbett, I'll be leaving in half an hour. Is there anything I can do for you before I leave?"

YOUR ANSWER

CORRECT ANSWER

Example II is better, because the nurse has left time to fulfill any of Mr. Tibbett's requests before she leaves.

87

Soon after the nurse goes off duty, Mr. Tibbett experiences severe pain in his stomach. He wants to ring for the nurse, but his call light or buzzer has fallen to the floor, and he cannot get out of bed to reach it. He has to call out for the nurse, and it is five minutes before anyone hears him and comes to help him. What should the nurse have done before she left Mr. Tibbett?

YOUR ANSWER

CORRECT ANSWER

She should have made sure that his call light or buzzer was secured within his reach.

88

The nurse usually states that she is leaving about half an hour before she actually leaves, and asks the patient if he has any requests that she can fulfill before she goes off duty. She should be sure that the patient's call light is within his reach. These actions carried out by the nurse are called *termination*.

(Go on to the next frame.)

89

You have been assigned to care for Mr. Robert Holmes until noon. It is now 11:30 A.M. You have completed Mr. Holmes' care, and he is resting comfortably in bed. He wants to read, and you feel you have met all of his immediate needs. As you leave to do your charting, you say to Mr. Holmes: (Quote yourself in one or two sentences.)

YOUR ANSWER

CORRECT ANSWER

"Mr. Holmes, I will be leaving at noon, which is in about half an hour. Is there anything more I can do for you between now and then?" (Pause while patient answers.) "Here is your call light. It is pinned to your pillowcase where you can reach it."

(Or equivalent response in which you include the three parts of termination.)

E. ORIENTATION TO TREATMENTS AND ACTIVITIES

BEHAVIORAL OBJECTIVE:

Before a patient has a treatment, the student states what it is, its purpose, frequency and duration. She also describes how it will feel and tells the patient his role in the treatment. (Frames 90–113)

90

Read all of the following examples, and state what common feeling you think that each of the people involved would have.

1. The electric power is cut off unexpectedly at 5:30 P.M. in New York City.

2. You are driving well within the legal speed limits on an expressway, and a policeman flags you over to the side of the road.

3. The telephone rings at 2:00 A.M.

4. A nurse, whom the patient knows, enters his room and pulls the curtain around his bed.

5. A doctor enters a patient's room with a strange looking device and says, "Would you please sit up and lean toward me?"

a. What is the common feeling?

YOUR ANSWER

CORRECT ANSWER

a. Anxiety, fear.

b. What is it in all these situations that induces this feeling?

YOUR ANSWER

CORRECT ANSWER

b. Uncertainty about what is happening.
(One doesn't know what to expect.)

91

Suppose instead that some of the previous situations were as follows:

1. The people in New York City knew that there had been a power failure at Niagara Falls.

2. You knew that your best friend would be at the airport briefly and would call you in the middle of the night.

3. The nurse told the patient, as she drew the curtain, that she was going to help him with his bath.

a. Would the same people have felt as fearful in these situations as in the previous situations?

YOUR ANSWER

CORRECT ANSWER

a. No.

b. Why?

YOUR ANSWER

CORRECT ANSWER

b. They knew what was happening.

92

These examples illustrate that when an event occurs unexpectedly, anxiety is likely to develop. This is likely to happen when the person does not understand the meaning of the event or perceives the possibility that what may happen will be threatening to him. Examples of the latter are situations where he may be deprived of something he needs, physically hurt, or embarrassed. Frequently, the hospitalized patient is subjected to diagnostic tests or therapeutic measures with which he is in part or totally unfamiliar. At times, events happen with which he may be familiar, but they happen at an unexpected time or in an unexpected way. An explanation should be given to the patient before any tests are administered. Frequently, this is the nurse's responsibility.

(Go on to the next frame.)

93

State what you would say to the patient in each of the following cases, if you were the approaching person.

1. You are an orderly, and you have to take Mr. Harrison to the barbershop in a wheel chair.

YOUR ANSWER

CORRECT ANSWER

1. "I'm Mr. X., the orderly. I'm here to take you to the barbershop, Mr. Harrison. Would you please get into the wheel chair?"

2. You are a nurse's aid and have to arrange some of the patient's personal items on his bedside stand in order to make room for a new bouquet of flowers.

YOUR ANSWER

CORRECT ANSWER

2. I'm Miss X. You have a new bouquet of flowers today. I need to move some of your things, so there's room for them."

3. You are a nurse and are caring for a patient who has a cast on his right leg from mid-thigh to mid-foot. You want to check his circulation, which you do by checking his toes for temperature and color. This is a routine kind of check.

YOUR ANSWER

CORRECT ANSWER

3. I'm Miss X. I just want to look at your toes and see if they're pink and warm. This is routine." (Or equivalent response.)

4. What have you tried to do in all of these cases?

YOUR ANSWER

CORRECT ANSWER

4. You told the patient what you were going to do before you did it.
You gave information which let the patient know what to expect.

94

When activities or treatments are scheduled for the patient, he frequently has questions about them. When an explanation of the treatment or activity is given to the patient, he has a better idea of what to expect, and anxiety is less likely to develop or to increase.

For example, imagine that you fractured your left elbow a month ago, and it had been immobilized in a cast until yesterday, when the cast was removed. At that time, the doctor told you that today you would begin to do range of motion exercises with your left arm.

What questions would you have about range of motion?

YOUR ANSWER

CORRECT ANSWER

These are some of the questions you might have.
1. What is range of motion?
2. What is the purpose? (What effect is range of motion supposed to have on my arm?)
3. How do I do it?
4. Will it hurt? (How will it feel?)
5. How long do I have to do range of motion?
6. How often do I have to do range of motion?

95

The questions that patients ask or think about vary somewhat in specific content. However, they can be generally categorized as follows, according to the kind of information that is sought:

Categories of Information

1. Description of the activity (In language that can be understood.)
2. Purpose or desired outcome of activity.
3. Patient's role in carrying out the activity. (How does he do it?)
4. An indication of how the activity will feel.
5. Frequency of the activity.
6. Duration of the activity.

(Go on to the next frame.)

96

Mr. Stone is going to have his gall bladder removed tomorrow.

The kardex states: three pHisoHex scrubs to the surgical area at intervals today, each scrub to last five minutes.

Miss Ames, the nurse, comes in to explain the scrub to him. Label each numbered, underlined statement in the explanation according to the kind of information the nurse is giving.

"Mr. Stone, the doctor wants you to give yourself three pHisoHex scrubs today.

1. This means that <u>your skin around the area of the operation is scrubbed with pHisoHex, a kind of soap</u>.

YOUR ANSWER

CORRECT ANSWER

1. Description of activity.

2. <u>This has to be done three times today: once this morning, once this afternoon, and once this evening, each time for five minutes.</u>

YOUR ANSWER

CORRECT ANSWER

2. Frequency and duration of activity.

3. <u>Of course, it won't hurt. It just feels cool, and your skin gets kind of dry.</u>

YOUR ANSWER

CORRECT ANSWER

3. Indication of how activity will feel.

4. <u>It removes as many of the bacteria from your skin as possible so that your skin will be clean before the operation.</u>

YOUR ANSWER

CORRECT ANSWER

4. Purpose of activity.

5. I'll bring you back a cup with pHisoHex and a cloth, and <u>you scrub this area</u> for five minutes. (Indicates with her hand the location and size of the area on the patient's abdomen.)

YOUR ANSWER

CORRECT ANSWER

5. Patient's role.

97

A nurse might orient the patient to an imposed task by answering his questions as they arise. But, sometimes, patients may have questions that they do not put directly to the nurse. If these questions remain unasked and unanswered, what feeling might the patient have?

YOUR ANSWER

CORRECT ANSWER

Anxiety, uneasiness.

98

How might the nurse attempt to prevent a patient's anxiety from developing or increasing about a procedure or treatment?

YOUR ANSWER

CORRECT ANSWER

By beginning a procedure or treatment with an explanation, rather than waiting for the patient to ask directly about it.

99

The next few frames deal more specifically with how the nurse orients the patient to a treatment or activity.

Read the following description of procedures that are given to the patient. Are these descriptions adequate and why?

1. The medical student enters the patient's unit and says, "Just sit up a minute, Mr. Jones. I'm going to do a little auscultation."

2. The nursing student enters the unit and says, "I want to check your vital signs."

3. The nurse comes in and says, "I'll be right back with the sphygmomanometer."

YOUR ANSWER

CORRECT ANSWER

No, because they use words that are unfamiliar to the patient.

100

The technical words just used have the following meanings:

1. Auscultation: listening to sounds other than voice sounds with an instrument other than the human ear (e.g., heart and lung sounds through a stethoscope).

2. Vital signs: blood pressure, pulse, and respiration.

3. Sphygmomanometer: device consisting of cuff, tubing, and pressure gauge, which is used to measure blood pressure.

Write what you would have said instead of:

1. "I'm going to do a little auscultation."

YOUR ANSWER

CORRECT ANSWER

1. "I want to listen to your heart or lungs with the stethoscope."

2. "I want to check your vital signs."

YOUR ANSWER

CORRECT ANSWER

2. "I want to take your pulse, respiration, and blood pressure."

3. "I'll be right back with the sphygmomanometer."

YOUR ANSWER

CORRECT ANSWER

3. "I'll be right back; I want to take your blood pressure."

101

It is important that the nurse explain the purpose of the treatment, because it is the patient's right to know, and he will be more likely to accept the treatment, if he understands how it may help him.

Below are listed several treatments for a patient who has pneumonia and knows his diagnosis. In Column A and in Column B are nurse's statements to the patient regarding the purpose of the treatments. In which column are the statements better and why?

Treatment	*Column A*	*Column B*
1. Penicillin 600,000 U. (IM) q. 12°.	1. This medication has been ordered to help you get well.	1. This medication will fight the organisms that are causing your pneumonia and help you get well.
2. Oxygen tent.	2. You are in the oxygen tent, because it is the doctor's order.	2. This will help you to breathe more easily.
3. Robitussin 1-2 tsp. (o) q. 4° p.r.n.	3. This is a common medication for people who have pneumonia.	3. This loosens and helps you to cough up the secretions that have accumulated in your lungs.

YOUR ANSWER

CORRECT ANSWER,

The statements in *Column B* are better, because they convey specific information about the effects of a treatment to the patient.

The answers in *Column A* simply state what the patient already knows: that the treatments he is receiving are for his pneumonia or have been ordered by the doctor.

102

Treatments are prescribed in the hope that the patient will be cured or the disease arrested. However, there can be no guarantee that the treatment will produce the desired effects. It is unethical and unkind to suggest that there will be a cure when there is no guarantee that there will be one. By describing the purpose of the treatment by its specific effects, this problem is more likely to be avoided.

For each of the examples of treatments below, select the correct nurse's statement for describing the purpose of the treatment to the patient.

Diagnosis	*Treatment*	*Choice of Nurse's Statements*	
1. Congestive heart failure	1. Digitoxin 0.1 mgm. (o) q.d.	1. a. This medication slows down the rate of your heart and helps it to pump more efficiently.	1. b. It will help your heart get better.
2. Fractured left femur eight weeks ago	2. Range of motion exercises to left leg for fifteen minutes q.i.d.	2. a. These exercises will help your leg get strong, so that you can walk as well as you used to.	2. b. These exercises should loosen up the muscles in your leg.
3. Asthma	3. Breathing into a machine that exerts positive pressure on the lungs, forcing open some of the congested and constricted bronchioles for ten minutes q.i.d.	3. a. When you do these breathing exercises with this machine, your asthma should improve.	3. b. When you do these breathing exercises with this machine, it should open up the air passageways in your lungs and help you to breathe easier.

YOUR ANSWER

CORRECT ANSWER

1. a.
2. b.
3. b.

103

Mrs. Ricks has psoriasis (a skin disease characterized by the formation of scaly red patches on the extensor surfaces of the body). Among her treatments every day are a bath with 30 ml. LCD (Liquor Carbonis Detergens: a coal tar prepartion which usually reduces redness and itching, and in the long run, it is hoped, will reduce the number and severity of the psoriatic lesions.)

You start the explanation by saying, "Mrs. Ricks, your bath today has some green soap in it."

What would you say to explain the purpose of the bath?

YOUR ANSWER

CORRECT ANSWER

"We hope that this will reduce the redness and itching of your skin."

(Or equivalent response in which you state the purpose in terms of specific effects.)

104

Mr. Sawyer had a wart removed from his right arm. He is to receive four warm compresses to the surgical site, each lasting for half an hour. They are to be given every four hours, starting at 10:00 A.M. Mr. Sawyer is up and around and frequently is off the ward visiting friends in other parts of the hospital or watching movies in the recreation room.

After you have described the compresses and told the purpose, what else do you say to Mr. Sawyer about them and why?

CORRECT ANSWER

"Mr. Sawyer, you'll have to do the compresses four times a day, each time for half an hour. The first one will be at 10:00 A.M., and then every four hours after that. You should be here at 10:00 A.M., 2:00 P.M., 6:00 P.M., and 10:00 P.M."

It lets him plan other activities, so that his regular activities will not conflict with the treatment.

105

Read the following examples:

1. The patient has to be there at the prescribed time to have a compress put on his right arm.

2. Post-operatively, the patient has to cough using his diaphragm and breathe deeply at least every two hours, in order to prevent fluid and mucus from accumulating in his lungs.

3. The diabetic patient should learn to give his own insulin.

These examples illustrate the importance of what factor in determining the effectiveness of the treatment?

YOUR ANSWER

CORRECT ANSWER

The patient's knowledge of the role he has in carrying out the treatment.

106

Mr. Roberts had right-sided chest surgery one week ago. The nurse notices that he does not elevate his right arm at all. She goes in to talk with him about exercising his right arm.

Nurse: "Mr. Roberts, it is important that you begin to exercise your right arm now, in order to loosen the muscles and help maintain the amount of motion you had in your arm before surgery. The way you exercise it is by trying to raise your right arm and by pointing your hand at the ceiling at least twice an hour. This may be somewhat painful at first, because you haven't moved your arm much since before the surgery. Begin by doing it gradually. Each time lift your arm a little higher than you did before, just past the point where it hurts."

The nurse returns in two hours to see how Mr. Roberts is doing with the exercise. The following conversation occurs.

Mr. Roberts: "I tried that exercise a couple of times, but whew! I just couldn't lift my arm; it seemed so heavy!"

Nurse: "Well, Mr. Roberts, you could use your left arm to help raise your right arm, or you could start by climbing your right fingers up the wall. Here, I'll show you."

What did the nurse fail to do on her first orientation?

YOUR ANSWER

CORRECT ANSWER

The nurse failed to tell him how he could do the exercise of his right arm, (i.e., his role in performing the task).

107

Read the following examples. What is the common element which the nurse fails to tell the patient to expect in each of the following situations?

1. The nurse gives an erythromycin injection which usually results in stinging. The patient says, "That really stings! I never had an injection that stung before. Is something the matter?"

2. The patient who just had surgery in his right eye complains of pain in his eye. The nurse brings back an ice pack that the doctor ordered and puts it on the patient's bandaged eye. The patient says, "Yi! That's sure cold! I jumped so when you put in on that I hope I didn't hurt my eye."

3. The patient just had his left elbow removed from a cast, where it had been for three weeks. He was to begin exercising it four times a day. The nurse saw him, after he had done it a couple of times, and the patient said, "It hurts worse since I started exercising it than it did when the doctor took the cast off. I'm worried about it!"

YOUR ANSWER

CORRECT ANSWER

She has failed to tell him how the treatment would feel.

108

These are good statements which could have been used to explain how the treatment in the preceding frame would feel.

1. "When the medicine is injected, it will sting for just a minute."

2. "I have an ice bag here for your eye. It will feel cold at first, but then you'll get used to it. Now, I will put it on."

3. "Since your arm has been in the cast, when you begin to exercise it, you will feel a dull pain in your muscles. This will probably last for a couple of days.

In each case, the nurse has described two pertinent factors regarding how the treatment will feel. What are they? In each case, answer in the general sense.

YOUR ANSWER

CORRECT ANSWER

1. Description of what will be felt.
2. Duration.

109

Anesthesia is used for very painful treatments. Therefore, treatments carried out without anesthesia rarely produce severe pain, although the patient may experience some degree of pain.

Which of the following statements is the most accurate description of a mildly painful procedure?
1. "This won't hurt a bit."
2. "You'll feel a dull pain for a few minutes."
3. "There will be an excruciating pain for a few minutes."

YOUR ANSWER

CORRECT ANSWER

2. "You'll feel a dull pain for a few minutes."

110

It is seldom accurate to describe the pain associated with a treatment as "excruciating," "unbearable," "horrible," or "knifelike."

Not only are such words inaccurate, but they are so extreme and frightening that the patient may feel more apprehensive than the treatment warrants. As a result he may refuse the treatment.

(Go on to the next frame.)

111

Here are some examples of the nurse orienting the patient as to how a treatment will feel.

1. Injection:
   "You will feel a sharp stabbing pain in your buttocks as I give this. It will only last a few seconds."
2. Removing bandage:
   "Mr. Jones, I'm going to rip off the bandage on your abdomen. It will probably feel like it's burning a little as I take it off, but I'll try to be fast."

State specifically:
a. What you think is wrong with these examples.

YOUR ANSWER

CORRECT ANSWER

a. The nurse uses emotionally charged words that depict the situation as being worse than it really is.

b. What effect might the examples have on the patient?

YOUR ANSWER

CORRECT ANSWER

b. The examples would probably cause increased anxiety, and the treatment might be refused.

112

Restate the preceding examples, so that they would not be expected to have these undesirable effects.

YOUR ANSWER

CORRECT ANSWER

1. "You'll feel a brief prick as I give you this injection."
2. "I am going to remove the bandage from your abdomen now. You'll probably feel a momentary pull or slight pressure while I do it."

(Or equivalent response, in which you describe the feeling as accurately as possible, avoiding the use of extreme or frightening words, and explaining approximately how long the feeling will last.)

113

Mr. Thomas is a forty-five year old man who will have his gall bladder removed tomorrow. You know that the physician has told him that post-operatively he will have to cough and deep breathe every two hours, and it would be a good idea for him to practice ahead of time.

You read the medical-nursing textbook which states: "two common pulmonary complications which may occur post-operatively are pneumonia and atelectasis (collapse or airless condition of part of the lung). A primary cause of these is incomplete aeration of the lungs with the formation of a mucus plug that may close one of the bronchi or bronchioles entirely. Since mucus is particularly thick post-operatively, and, therefore, likely to accumulate in the lungs, it is important that the patient cough at least every two hours for two or three minutes and adequately expand his lungs at intervals. Many patients do not carry out these activities because of the pain involved and pressure felt on the stitches. However, the nurse can help the patient by 'splinting' (holding to prevent movement) the incision, using a pillow, towel, or her hands to apply moderate pressure. This will support the incision. It is important that the patient cough from his diaphragm and not just in his throat."

What do you *say* to Mr. Thomas about the coughing and deep breathing?

(Report the actual words you would use.)

YOUR ANSWER

CORRECT ANSWER

Your orientation may vary in words, but you should have included the following:

a. Description of task.

b. Purpose.

c. Patient's role.

d. How will it feel.

e. Frequency and duration.

Here is an example of what you might have said.

"Mr. Thomas, after your operation the doctor wants you to *(a) cough and breathe deeply (e) for two or three minutes every two hours. This is (b) so that you will expand your lungs and get air into all parts of them. You will have a tendency to have more mucus in your lungs after surgery, so it is especially important that you cough, in order to remove it.* I realize *(d) that it will be painful* at the beginning. I will help you by using a towel to put pressure on your incision, so it won't hurt so much. *(c) It is important that you take a deep breath before you cough. Cough from your lungs, not just in your throat.* Let's try it a few times right now."

BEHAVIORAL OBJECTIVE:

The student records administered treatments correctly in the nursing notes. (Frames 114–118)

114

After the nurse has carried out the procedure or treatment, she charts that it was done in the nursing notes. The charting of treatments in the nursing notes is a permanent record showing that ordered treatments have been carried out. Read the examples below, and then state what kinds of information the nurse puts in the nursing notes.

1. Miss Joan Smith carries out a treatment at 10:00 A.M. on June fourth and charts it as follows: "Warm saline soak to left elbow for 20" q.i.d. 10:00 A.M./J.S."

2. Miss Sarah Brown charts a treatment she carried out at 9:00 A.M. on June fourth as follows: "Crude coal tar to lesions on back and extremities q.d. 9:00 A.M./S.B."

3. Miss Betsy Moffett charts a treatment she carried out at 10:00 A.M. on June fourth as follows: "Range of motion to right leg for 15" t.i.d. 10:00 A.M./B.M."

YOUR ANSWER

CORRECT ANSWER

Kinds of information included in charting treatments or procedures:

1. What the treatment or procedure is.

2. Where it is to be applied.

3. For how long it should be applied (where appropriate).

4. How often it is ordered.

5. What time it was applied.

6. The initials of the person who applied it.

115

Miss Nancy Burns is caring for Mrs. Rock. Mrs. Rock's kardex reads:
"Sterile dressing to lesion on left ankle t.i.d."
Write down what Miss Burns would put on Mrs. Rock's nursing notes after she carried out the treatment at 9:00 A.M.

YOUR ANSWER

CORRECT ANSWER

Sterile dressing applied to lesion on left ankle t.i.d. 9:00 A.M./N.B.

116

When the same treatment is to be given more than once during the day, the nurse needs only to write the time and her initials after the original charting. Using the same examples from a previous frame, note how treatments after the first one are recorded.

1. Warm saline soak to left elbow for 20" q.i.d. 10:00 A.M./J.S. 2:00 P.M./L.R., 6:00 P.M./O.P., 10:00 P.M./N.Q.

2. Range of motion to right leg for 15" t.i.d. 10:00 A.M./B.M., 2:00 P.M./L.R., 6:00 P.M./O.P.

(Go on to the next frame.)

117

Besides charting that the treatment was done, the nurse should also write in the nursing notes how the treated area looked and how the patient responded to the treatment. Look at the examples below, and fill in the last example of what the nurse might put in the nursing notes.

Treatment	Patient Response and Appearance of Area	Nursing Notes
1. Warm compress to IV site on left forearm 20" q.i.d.	1. IV site is purplish-green in color and only slightly swollen.	1. IV site appeared purplish-green and slightly edematous.
2. Postural drainage 15" t.i.d. after meals.	2. The patient complains the whole time she is doing it, "I can't breathe! I can't cough up anything, because I feel like I'm suffocating!" She usually stops after five minutes and does not cough up any mucus.	2. Patient only able to carry out postural drainage for five minutes at 10:00 A.M. States, "I can't breathe!" during exercise. Her cough during this time is non-productive.

Treatment	*Patient Response and Appearance of Area*	*Nursing Notes*
3. Range of motion to right arm 15" t.i.d.	3. The patient has no difficulty with any of the exercises, except that she cannot raise her arm above shoulder height without experiencing a sharp pain in her shoulder. This pain is relieved after administration of Darvon, and the patient is able to continue the exercises.	YOUR ANSWER

CORRECT ANSWER

During performance of range of motion exercises, the patient reported a sharp pain in her shoulder when she extended her arm above shoulder height. Darvon was administered. Treatment continued after patient reported relief from pain.

118

When the physician reads what the nurse has written in the nursing notes about the treatment, it helps him to decide if the treatment should be continued, and if he should change his orders to make the treatment more effective. For example, he might order a pain medication to be given to the person who is doing range of motion exercises.

(Go on to the next frame.)

119

When the nurse carries out a treatment and observes the patient's reaction to it, she decides if there are ways she can increase the effectiveness of the treatment. For example, she may find a more comfortable position for the patient during a treatment, or she may administer a p.r.n. pain medication prior to beginning a treatment. The things she learns can guide other nurses in caring for the patient and are recorded in the Guides to Nursing Management.

(Go on to the next frame.)

120

Look at the examples below and fill in the missing information.

Treatment	Patient Response	Nursing Notes	Guides To Nursing Management
1. Range of motion to right arm 15 minutes t.i.d.	1. The patient has no difficulty with any of the exercises except that she cannot raise her arm above shoulder height without experiencing a sharp pain in her shoulder. This pain is relieved after administration of Darvon and the patient is able to continue the exercises.	1. During performance of range of motion exercises the patient reported a sharp pain in her shoulder when she extended her arm above shoulder height. Darvon was administered. Treatment continued after patient reported relief from pain.	YOUR ANSWER
			CORRECT ANSWER
			1. Guides: Patient performs exercises more comfortably when Darvon is administered prior to range of motion.
2. Cough and deep breathe q. 30.	2. The patient says, "I feel like I'm going to pull out the stitches when I cough and deep breathe. It really hurts!" When a bath blanket is pressed tightly against the incision the patient has less difficulty carrying out the treatment.	YOUR ANSWER	YOUR ANSWER
		CORRECT ANSWER	CORRECT ANSWER
		2. Nursing notes: Bath blanket held tightly against incision while patient coughed and breathed deeply.	2. Guides: Patient coughs and deep breathes with less pain when his incision is splinted with a bath blanket.

F. MODIFIED ORIENTATION TO TREATMENTS AND ACTIVITIES

121

We have just said that the nurse orients the patient to a task or treatment. However, when a patient is given the same treatment repeatedly over a period of days or weeks, how might he be expected to feel if each time the treatment is carried out the nurse gave full information concerning the treatment, purpose, duration, desired outcome, and degree of pain to be expected?

YOUR ANSWER

CORRECT ANSWER

Bored or irritated.

122

The nurse should inform other nurses that the patient has been oriented. What he understands about the task, and what parts of it, if any, he needs help with should also be charted. This communication occurs by way of the kardex in the "Guides to Nursing Management" section. In this way the patient may be spared repeated explanations of the same task.

For example:

Guides to Nursing Management.

1. Patient can do full range of motion on all extremeities. He needs help with his left leg.

(Go on to the next frame.)

123

Read the following interaction in which Miss Bridges is orienting Mr. Bay to a new treatment. Write down what the nurse would record on the "Guides to Nursing Management." Mr. Bay's kardex card reads: Isuprel nebulizer (an atomizer) with 2 cc. of Isuprel 15" q.i.d.

Miss Bridges enters Mr. Bay's unit with the nebulizer containing 2 cc. of Isuprel.

Mr. Bay: "Hello, Miss Bridges."

Miss Bridges: "Hello, Mr. Bay. It's time for you to breathe using this nebulizer. It works like an atomizer."

Mr. Bay: "Oh, yes. The doctor said I would have to do this."

Miss Bridges: "You'll have to do it four times a day, for fifteen minutes each time. As you breathe in the mist from the nebulizer it helps to liquefy some of the mucus you have in your lungs, so that it will be easier for you to cough it up. I'll show you how it works. (Shows the patient and watches him do it.) Can you breathe more deeply, so that the mist goes farther into your lungs?"

Mr. Bay: "Oh, I'll try. I have to concentrate so hard on breathing in when I squeeze the nebulizer, that sometimes I forget to breathe deeply."

Miss Bridges: "Well, the mist is more effective if you can breathe deeply. Perhaps, each time you do it for the next day or so, one of the nurses could watch you for a few minutes and see that you're breathing deeply."

Mr. Bay: "That would be fine, just as a reminder."

YOUR ANSWER

CORRECT ANSWER

"Guides to Nursing Management":

Patient oriented to using the Isuprel nebulizer. He needs to be reminded to breathe deeply; therefore, the nurse should see that he is doing this each time he uses the nebulizer.

124

When it is written on the kardex that the patient has been oriented to a task or a treatment and his capabilities have been listed, the nurse assumes that what is written is accurate. She does not need to reorient the patient, unless there is some change in the treatment.

(Go on to the next frame.)

125

However, when there is nothing written on the "Guides to Nursing Management," the nurse cannot assume that the patient has received the orienting information, even though he has performed the task. The nurse must assess how much of the orienting information the patient has understood and what his capabilities are in performing the task. Then, it is the nurse's responsibility to record the patient's degree of understanding and his capabilities in performing the task on the "Guides to Nursing Management."

(Go on to the next frame.)

126

Consider the following example.

Miss Brickner is caring for Mrs. Rogers. According to the kardex card, Mrs. Rogers is to exercise her left leg with a Banno Skate for fifteen minutes three times a day. Miss Brickner does not know whether Mrs. Rogers has ever done this type of exercise before. Therefore, she asks her if she has. Mrs. Rogers says, "No."

What should Miss Brickner do?

YOUR ANSWER

CORRECT ANSWER

She should orient Mrs. Rogers to the exercise with the Banno Skate. After Mrs. Rogers has exercised, the nurse should record in the "Guides to Nursing Management" that Mrs. Rogers was oriented and performed the task.

127

Now suppose that when Miss Brickner asked Mrs. Rogers if she had ever exercised with a Banno Skate, Mrs. Rogers said, "Yes, I have."

Remembering that the nurse is responsible for the accuracy of what she records, this is an example of how Miss Brickner could proceed.

Miss Brickner: "I will get the board up on the bed for you and strap the skate on. Do you have any questions about this exercise?"

Mrs. Rogers: "I can't remember exactly how long I should do it."

Miss Brickner: "For about fifteen minutes three times a day."

Mrs. Rogers: "Oh, yes, now I remember. I certainly hope it will loosen the muscles in my leg! They seem so tight after being in traction for two months."

Miss Brickner: "Yes, that is why you're doing the exercises." (Nurse watches her perform the exercises for a few minutes.) "It looks like you are doing them correctly. I'll be back in a few minutes and help you take the skate off."

(Go on to the next frame.)

128

Here is another example. Read it, and then answer the question below.

Miss Bates is assigned to care for Mr. Fisher. The big toe on his right foot is infected.

His kardex reads: Warm saline compress to right big toe for 20" q.i.d. followed by dry sterile dressing.

There is nothing about the task written on the "Guides to Nursing Management." Miss Bates asks Mr. Fisher if he has ever done the compress and applied the dressing, and he says, "Yes."

What does Miss Bates do and say now?

YOUR ANSWER

CORRECT ANSWER

She would either watch him do the compress or talk to him about it, giving him information about aspects that he does not mention and correcting any misconceptions he may have had. Then she writes the appropriate comments on the "Guides to Nursing Management."

129

Below is an example in dialogue of how Miss Bates' conversation with Mr. Fisher might have gone.

Miss Bates: "I will bring you the equipment and help you get started. Is there any kind of equipment that you prefer?"

Mr. Fisher: "I like one of those kidney shaped bowls. My foot fits in it better. Otherwise, just bring in what you think I need."

Miss Bates: "All right." (Brings in equipment and helps Mr. Fisher.) "Do you have any questions about the soak or putting on the dressing?"

Mr. Fisher: "Could I keep the bottle of saline here and change the saline after ten minutes or so? It gets kind of cold after twenty minutes, and the doctor said it should be warm to improve the circulation and help get rid of the infection."

Miss Bates: "Yes, you can keep the saline now. You know you're to do this four times a day. Someone will bring you a new warmed bottle each time. I'll be back in twenty minutes to watch you put on the dressing and see that you know how to do it."

Mr. Fisher: "Okay. Thanks."

Write down what Miss Bates would write in the "Guides to Nursing Management."

YOUR ANSWER

CORRECT ANSWER

"Guides to Nursing Management":

Patient has been oriented to the compress on his right big toe. He prefers to use a kidney basin and to keep the bottle of saline there during the compress.

130

In the preceding frames, you have seen how the nurse assesses what the patient knows about a treatment or a task. In these examples, as well as in any others, when the patient states that he knows about a treatment or a task, the nurse still has to make certain that he knows the six parts of the orientation.

1. What the treatment is.
2. Purpose of the treatment.
3. How it will feel.
4. Patient's role in carrying out the treatment.
5. Duration.
6. Frequency.

(Go on to the next frame.)

131

The nurse should give orienting information about herself or about the imposed task, so that the patient will have the opportunity to develop more realistic expectations about what the nurse will be doing for him and about what will be happening to him. However, it is always possible that the patient will not understand the orienting information, or that he may act as though he understands it, and a few days later ask questions that have already been answered.

(Go on to the next frame.)

132

When patients are highly anxious, they may not understand explanations. The patient may be preoccupied with other matters, such as impending surgery or wondering if he is going to recover. Often, just being in the hospital itself is anxiety-producing. This may lead to the patient not understanding what is explained to him. Therefore, it may be necessary for the nurse to repeat the explanation at some later time.

(Go on to the next frame.)

G. OFFERING CHOICE TO THE PATIENT

BEHAVIORAL OBJECTIVES:

When the medical regimen does not allow the patient a choice, the student does not offer one.
When choices are allowed, the student finds out patient's preferences and takes direct action or communicates with appropriate personnel in order to permit choice. (Frames 133–144)

133

When the patient is in the hospital, the physician orders treatments. As the nurse carries them out, she also makes observations. In the first part of the program, you learned how to use the resources to find out the physician's orders. In some cases, the physician specifies the exact time and manner in which treatments must be carried out. In other cases, the nurse has more latitude in carrying out the treatments and observations and may consider the patient's preferences and her own schedule.

(Go on to the next frame.)

134

The following physician's orders are written on your patient's kardex. In each case, specify the letters of the action or actions that carry out the physician's orders appropriately.

Physician's Orders	*Nursing Actions*
1. Force fluids 3000 cc./day.	1. a. Patient drinks one glass (250 cc.) of water every hour, while awake.
	b. Patient drinks one glass of grape juice every hour, while awake.
	c. Patient drinks two glasses of liquid at each meal and one glass every two hours, while awake.

YOUR ANSWER

CORRECT ANSWER

1. a, b, c.

2. Sit in chair 20" b.i.d.	2. a. Patient sits in chair 20" to eat breakfast and 20" in midafternoon.
	b. Patient sits in chair for 20" in midmorning and 20" in the evening when he has visitors.
	c. Patient sits up for 40" to eat lunch.

YOUR ANSWER

CORRECT ANSWER

2. a, b.

3. Change patient's position q. 2°.	3. a. Patient's position is changed q. 2°.
	b. Patient's position is changed at 7:00 A.M. Nurse comes in at 9:00 A.M. and finds the patient sleeping. She decides to let him sleep and not change his position until he wakes up.
	c. Nurse comes in to change patient's position, and he says, "I'm comfortable as I am." She lets him stay that way and does not change his position.

YOUR ANSWER

CORRECT ANSWER

3. a.

135

Look again at Mr. Willoughby's kardex. Here are two of the physician's orders for Mr. Willoughby:
1. Encourage fluids to 3000 cc.
2. Cough and turn q. 2°.

Consider both the requirements of these orders and the patient's preferences. Describe how you would carry them out.

YOUR ANSWER

CORRECT ANSWER

1. I would give him his preference about enough grape juice, apple juice, and water, so that he would have 3000 cc.

2. Cough and turn q. 2°. I would use a bath blanket around his chest and over the incision to hold his side when he coughs. (Patient's preferences found in "Guides to Nursing Management.")

136

Look at Miss Groom's kardex. The physician has ordered "Special skin care: cleanse carefully, and rub with Dermassage lotion.

Consider both the requirements of this order and the patient's preference, and describe how you would carry it out.

YOUR ANSWER

CORRECT ANSWER

Cleanse her skin with her own soap, and rub with Dermassage lotion.

137

The preceding examples have shown you when and how a treatment may be modified to be consistent with the patient's preferences. The knowledge that will enable you to determine when there is latitude and the extent of the latitude you will gain throughout your nursing studies. It is important in nursing not to offer the patient a choice if you cannot abide by his decision. However, the nurse should offer the patient a choice whenever it is possible according to the medical or nursing therapies.

In the next section of the program, we will give you some examples of how the principles of choice may be applied.

(Go on to the next frame.)

138

Look at the following example, and describe what went wrong.

Mother: "Patty, it's eight o'clock. Don't you want to go to sleep now?"

Patty: "No, I think I'd rather watch the rest of Lassie."

Mother: (Firmly.) "Young lady, it's eight o'clock. You're going to sleep right now!"

Patty: (Crying.) "But you asked me if I wanted to go to sleep, and I told you. I don't want to go to sleep! I want to watch Lassie!"

Mother: (Angrily.) "Stop being impossible! Go to bed!"

Patty: (Cries.)

YOUR ANSWER

CORRECT ANSWER

The mother implied that Patty had a choice about going to bed, when she had no choice at all.

139

Mr. Whitman is a newly diagnosed diabetic patient who will be discharged this afternoon. It is necessary for Miss Adams, the nurse, to talk with him about his diet before he goes home. Read the example below, and state Miss Adams' error in approaching Mr. Whitman.

Miss Adams: "May I sit down and talk with you for a few minutes about your diet, Mr. Whitman?"

Mr. Whitman: "No, I don't want to talk about it right now."

YOUR ANSWER

CORRECT ANSWER

Miss Adams implied that Mr. Whitman had a choice about talking with her.

140

What could Miss Adams have said instead of, "May I sit down and talk with you?"

YOUR ANSWER

CORRECT ANSWER

She should have sat down and then said, "Since you're going home this afternoon, I need to talk with you for a few minutes regarding your diet, Mr. Whitman. Now seems to be the best time."

(Or any equivalent response which does not give him a choice.)

141

Sometimes, doctor's orders permit some degree of choice to the patient, but there are restrictions or boundaries on that choice. Here are two examples of the nurse and the patient talking. In which example is the nurse more effective? Why?

Example I

Miss Jones: "Hello, Mrs. Webb. Here is your menu for tomorrow. I want you to select some things that you will want to eat. Circle the ones that you want."

Mrs. Webb: "I'll have some spaghetti, a green salad, and some ice cream for lunch."

Miss Jones: "I'm afraid you won't be able to eat the spaghetti, Mrs. Webb. You're on a controlled diet for starches. Why don't you pick out something else?"

Mrs. Webb: "I don't really know what the starches are. I don't know how to choose a menu."

Example II

Miss Jones: "I'd like you to select the foods that you want to eat for tomorrow. Here's your menu. Just circle the foods that you want. Remember that you are not to eat much starch. I've crossed out the items on the menu that you cannot have. So, go ahead and circle any of the others that you'd like."

Miss Webb: "Okay. I kind of hate to miss out on the spaghetti, but there are some other good things here. I guess I'll have a steak, a green salad, and maybe some of the peaches."

YOUR ANSWER

CORRECT ANSWER

Example II, because she describes the restrictions on the patient's choice before asking her to make a decision.

142

Here is a different example. In which example is the nurse more effective and why?

Example I

Miss Jones: "Mrs. Webb, it's time for you to bathe now. I've arranged to have the shower available for you for the next fifteen minutes."

Fifteen minutes later Mrs. Webb returns.

Mrs. Webb: "Well, that was nice, but I really wish I could've taken a bath. I always take a bath at home, and I really don't like showers."

Example II

Miss Jones: "Good morning, Mrs. Webb. It's time for you to bathe now. Would you prefer a shower or a bath?"

Mrs. Webb: "I think I'd like to take a bath."

Miss Jones: "I'll go and see if the room is ready."

YOUR ANSWER

CORRECT ANSWER

Example II, because the nurse presents choices that are available to the patient.

143

To summarize:

1. If you cannot abide by the patient's decision, do not offer a choice.
2. Set the limits *before* the discussion with the patient.
3. If alternatives *are* available, tell the patient what they are.
4. Remember that offering a choice to the patient is governed by the medical and nursing therapies that are planned for the patient.

(Go on to the next frame.)

144

You are assigned to care for Mrs. Fulton. Look at her data to refresh your memory, if you wish.

It is now 10:00 A.M. You have just finished bathing Mrs. Fulton. Suddenly, you realize that you have not offered her any fluids to drink this morning. She has had no water since shortly after breakfast.

What do you say to Mrs. Fulton? Why do you state it the way you do?

YOUR ANSWER

CORRECT ANSWER

It's time that you drink some fluids, Mrs. Fulton. What kind of drink would you prefer: water, grape juice, or pineapple juice?"

(Or equivalent response.)

You state it this way, so you do not give her a choice about drinking but do give her a choice about what to drink.

Part III

COMMUNICATION SKILLS

A. INTRODUCTION

145

Each time the nurse helps the patient to take care of some of his physical needs or just talks with him, she finds out more about what he is like as a unique individual. There are communication skills which enable the nurse to better understand the patient (and to help the patient understand her). We will present them in the next section of this program. As you read this section, keep in mind that, although skills are useful, there must be an underlying desire on the part of one individual, the nurse, to relate to another individual, the patient, as a unique person.

(Go on to the next frame.)

B. UNDERSTANDING WHAT THE PATIENT MEANS

BEHAVIORAL OBJECTIVES:

When the patient expresses feeling, the student encourages him to continue through reflecting feeling, raising open-ended questions, or in some other way giving the patient the opportunity to express his feelings and/or begin the process of problem solving. (Frames 146–166)

When statements or questions made by a patient are not sufficiently clear to imply specific nursing action, the student will elicit further information and take action only when the patient's meaning has been clarified. For example:

    a. When the patient resists an ordered treatment. (See frames 175–186)
    b. When the patient criticizes the staff or his treatment. (See frames 167–174)
    c. When the patient reports pain or discomfort in vague or ambiguous words. (See frames 146–166)
    d. When the patient makes vague, indefinite statements or uses pronouns without referents. (See frames 156–157)

146

One general principle is that *communication from the patient will be encouraged, if the nurse understands the meaning of what the patient says and conveys her understanding to him.* Consider the following short interaction: (1) Does the nurse convey to the patient that she understands what he means? (2) If not, how might she have done this?

Patient: "I'm a terrible bother, aren't I?"

Nurse: "You're not a bother, Mrs. Clifford. I enjoy being your nurse."

Patient: "I didn't mean to *you;* I'm a bother to my family."

YOUR ANSWER

CORRECT ANSWER

1. No, she indicates that she misunderstood the meaning of his question.

2. She might have found out specifically what the patient meant, rather than drawing premature conclusions.

147

When patients raise questions about problems they have or decisions they must make, the immediate response may be to give advice, to urge the patient to follow the doctors orders, or to suggest to the patient that he should not even be thinking about a question. Imagine yourself as the patient in each of these situations. Would you feel like expressing yourself any further after the nurse's response? Why?

Patient:	*Nurse:*
1. "I can't decide whether to have surgery or not."	1. "I'm sure the doctor knows best."
2. "My family doesn't seem to understand about my illness."	2. "They may seem not to, but I'm sure they do."
3. "I just can't see how I'll be able to follow my new diet when I go home."	3. "It's important for your health that you do."
4. "I feel depressed about my illness."	4. "Oh, but you're doing just fine!"

YOUR ANSWER

CORRECT ANSWER

No, the nurse has not encouraged the patient to provide any additional description of the problem. Indeed, her remarks have glossed over the patient's concerns.

148

Communication, like other behaviors, is more likely to continue if it is rewarded or, at least, not punished. If the nurse states or implies that the patient's statements are unworthy or inappropriate, she will tend to cut off communication. For example, do you think the patient would continue his discussion with the nurses in the following situations? Why or why not?

Patient:	*Nurse:*
1. "I'm a little afraid of my appendectomy tomorrow."	1. "The doctors are competent, and appendectomies are rather simple operations."
2. "It's funny, but I feel blue today."	2. "It's so nice outside. You'll probably feel better if you can see outside. I'll open the curtains."
3. "I feel very isolated in the hospital."	3. "But your wife has been coming every day!"

YOUR ANSWER

CORRECT ANSWER

Probably not. The nurse has in each case denied that the feeling is warranted. She has punished his attempts to express himself.

149

In the previous frame the patients have described feelings they are experiencing. The nurse might respond by suggesting to the patient that he tell her more about how he is feeling. Interest in the patient's feeling without criticism can be conveyed in another way. She may indicate that she is aware of his feelings by restating or describing briefly to him what she perceives him to be feeling. This is called reflecting feeling. Consider how you would feel in the following situations. Would you feel your friend was aware of your feeling? Would you be likely to talk more about it?

You:	*Your Friend:*
"I could just scream at Arthur!"	"You sound really angry with him!"
"I'm awfully scared of that math exam."	"You're afraid of not doing as well as you'd like?"
"I feel like I'm going to cry."	"You look sad."

YOUR ANSWER

CORRECT ANSWER

We think so. Your friend recognized your feeling. You would probably continue to talk about it.

150

How might you respond to each of the patient's statements below? In your answers indicate to the patient that you are aware of his feeling without implying that it is inappropriate.

Patient:	*Your Response:*
1. "I'm a little afraid of my appendectomy tomorrow."	**YOUR ANSWER**
	CORRECT ANSWER
	1. "You're uneasy about the operation?"
2. "It's funny, but I feel blue today."	**YOUR ANSWER**
	CORRECT ANSWER
	2. "You seem downhearted."
3. "I feel very isolated in the hospital."	**YOUR ANSWER**
	CORRECT ANSWER
	3. "You feel lonely here." (Or equivalent responses.)

151

When the patient is talking and you occasionally respond by nodding or looking at him with interest, what does this indicate to him?

YOUR ANSWER

CORRECT ANSWER

That you understand what he is saying and are waiting for him to continue.

152

Frequently, by talking with the patient and exploring what he means, the nurse is able to take direct nursing action, i.e., (1) finding out the patient's reasons for resisting a treatment and then modifying the treatment accordingly; (2) eliciting a more specific description when a patient complains of pain, so that she can apply appropriate relief measures.

At other times, although there is no specific action that the nurse can take on the basis of what she finds out, talking with the patient serves a useful purpose. It helps him to explore his own feelings and reactions.

(Go on to the next frame.)

153

In earlier segments of the program we developed the use of written resources to provide information that directs and facilitates effective patient care. The patient is also a resource of information which may or may not imply action. For example:

Patient's Statements	*Implied Action*
1. "I feel very tired. Would you please turn off the radio so that I can sleep?"	1. Turn off the radio.
2. "The bath water is too cold. Would you warm it up a bit?"	2. Warm bath water.
3. "I have a lot of pain in my leg again. May I have another pain pill?"	3. Assuming doctor's orders permit, give patient ordered medication for pain.

(Go on to the next frame.)

154

Frequently, the patient will say something that is unclear or subject to more than one interpretation. In this instance what action is implied for the nurse? Why?
1. "I don't like the food in the hospital."
2. "I don't feel very well today."
3. "I'd rather you didn't change my bandage."

YOUR ANSWER

CORRECT ANSWER

No clear action is implied, because the patient's statements are unclear. (You may have anticipated us and said, "Find out specifically what the patient means." If so, good!)

155

When the patient says something that is unclear or could be interpreted in more than one way, the nurse should encourage the patient to clarify his meaning. Only when the patient's meaning is clear can the nurse take appropriate action.

One method for encouraging further communication is illustrated in the nurse's responses below. All of the nurse's responses illustrate one method for eliciting futher description: Use of the open-ended question or statement.

Statement	*Response*
1. "I don't want to do that!"	1. "You don't?", "Oh?"
2. "This has been a dismal day."	2. "What happened?", "Tell me about it."
3. "I don't like this hospital!"	3. "What do you mean?", "You don't?"
4. "I don't want to go home."	4. "You don't?", "Would you tell me more about that?"

156

Another method of eliciting further description is used when patients' statements are not clear, because pronouns are used without a clear referent. For example, the patient may refer to "him," "they," or "this" without making it clear to the nurse about whom or of what he is speaking. Suppose you were the nurse to whom each of the following statements was made:

A. *What might you say in response to each statement?*

  1. "They said I could go home tomorrow."

YOUR ANSWER

CORRECT ANSWER

  1. Who are they?

  2. "He said I should spend more time out of bed."

YOUR ANSWER

CORRECT ANSWER

  2. Who said that you should?

  3. "They really get on my nerves."

YOUR ANSWER

CORRECT ANSWER

    3. Who do?

    4. "It's getting me down."

YOUR ANSWER

CORRECT ANSWER

    4. Tell me what you mean by "it"?

    5. "This is the last straw."

YOUR ANSWER

CORRECT ANSWER

    5. What happened?

    6. "I guess I'd better not worry about that."

YOUR ANSWER

CORRECT ANSWER

    6. What do you mean by that?

B. *What are you attempting to do in your responses?*

YOUR ANSWER

CORRECT ANSWER

    Attempting to identify the referent for the indefinite pronoun in order to understand what the patient means.

157

    Identifying the referent for indefinite pronouns serves to clarify the meaning of ambiguous statements which are made by the patient. The patient may use vague phrases or statements which may appropriately be dealt with in similar fashion. For example, in each of these responses, the nurse has attempted to get the patient to specify what he means.

Patient's Statement:	*Nurse's Response:*
"I'm in a funny mood today."	"What do you mean by 'funny mood'?"
"For a long time now, I've been anxious."	"When did this start?"
"I wish I could understand what my doctor meant."	"What did he say?"

(Go on to the next frame.)

158

By clarifying a patient's statement which does not clearly suggest action, you may gain information that will help you decide upon appropriate action. For example:

Patient: "I don't want my breakfast today."

Nurse: "You don't want to eat your breakfast?"

Possible Next Responses	*Nursing Action*
1. "I just don't like eggs. Could I have something else?"	1. Obtain other food permitted by patient's diet.
2. "I feel too queasy to eat."	2. Further exploration might lead the nurse to offer medication, inform the physician, etc.
3. "My headache is so severe that I don't want to eat."	3. Provide pain medication if ordered by physician, or contact physician to get an order for pain medication.

(Go on to the next frame.)

159

When the patient is encouraged to go on, his meaning may immediately become clear or it my not. If the patient's response remains ambiguous, the nurse encourages him in a nondirective way to go on again. However, if the patient mentions something more specific, the nurse should encourage him to elaborate upon this. Suppose that the patient says, "This has been a dismal day." and you have responded, "Go on." Below in the column on the left are different responses that the patient might make. In the column on the right are the comments that the nurse might make next.

Different Responses	*Nurse Comments*
1. "Maybe it's just me."	1. "Oh?"
2. "My wife won't be coming to see me until this weekend."	2. "You won't be able to see her for a few days?"
3. "The doctor told me I might have to have surgery."	3. "Tell me about what he said."
4. "My leg has been aching all day long."	4. "Can you describe what kind of ache it is and exactly where you have it?"
5. "I always like to read the *New York Times* in the morning, and it hadn't come in yet when I went down to get it."	5. "I'll call to see if it has come in yet."

(Go on to the next frame.)

160

Here is an interaction that might follow when the patient says, "This has been a dismal day." Notice that as the patient is better able to define the problem, the nurse's response becomes increasingly specific. The problem soon becomes apparent to both the patient and the nurse, and then a nursing action, if indicated, can be taken.

Mr. Wilke: "This has been a dismal day."

Mrs. Garner: "Go on."

Mr. Wilke: "My leg has been aching all day long."

Mrs. Garner: "Can you describe what kind of ache it is and exactly where you have it?"
Mr. Wilke: "It's like the pain I had yesterday. My knee throbs."
Mrs. Garner: "I remember that you were given some pain medication yesterday. Did it help you then?"
Mr. Wilke: "Yes."
Mrs. Garner: "Would you like some now?"
Mr. Wilke: "I thought I could get by without it, but I guess I'd better have some."
Mrs. Garner: "I'll be right back with it."

(Go on to the next frame.)

161

Look at the examples of statements by the patient listed below, and write one response that the nurse might give in each instance.

 1. Patient: "I had a lot of pain last night."

YOUR ANSWER

CORRECT ANSWER

 1. Please describe the pain; or what was the pain like?

 2. Patient: "I'm not going to do that soak."

YOUR ANSWER

CORRECT ANSWER

 2. You don't want to do the soak? or What's the matter?

 3. Patient: "I have a headache."

YOUR ANSWER

CORRECT ANSWER

 3. Would you tell me about your headache? or Describe how it feels.

 4. Patient: "I'd like to sleep all day."

YOUR ANSWER

CORRECT ANSWER

 4. You would? All day?
(Or equivalent responses in which you did not draw inferences beyond what the patient had specifically stated.)

(Go on to the next frame.)

162

The nurse should make it clear to the patient that one of her goals is to clarify meaning for herself and help him clarify meaning for himself. She implies in their dialogue the following: "Do I understand you?", "Correct me if I'm wrong.", "Is this what you mean?" She should not draw inferences as though they were definitive and not subject to revision.

Rewrite the examples below so that they satisfy the criteria stated above:

	YOUR ANSWER
1. "It's very clear to me that . . ."	1.
2. "You believe that this is so."	2.
3. "It's obvious that you're mad at the world."	3.

CORRECT ANSWER

1. "From what you say it seems that . . ."
2. "You appear to think that this is so."
3. "You seem to be angry."

Your answers should imply that your interpretations are tentative rather than final.

163

In the preceding frames we have discussed two techniques:

1. Making increasingly specific responses as the patient's meaning becomes more clear.
2. Drawing inferences in a tentative form.

Both these techniques allow you to confirm that you have an accurate view of how the patient is experiencing his situation. When you confirm this, you are validating your impressions with the patient.

(Go on to the next frame.)

164

Often when the nurse asks the patient to go on or to clarify a vague statement, the patient will respond by telling the nurse what he means. However, there are times when the patient might not go on, because (1) the idea is so vague in his own mind that he cannot express it any more clearly, (2) he may have changed his mind and not wish to talk about it with anyone, (3) he may prefer to talk to someone else about the situation. If further discussion indicates that the patient does not want to continue the topic, the nurse should respect his wish.

(Go on to the next frame.)

165

Suppose that the patient has said, "I didn't sleep well last night." The nurse would say, "Tell me more about that." Look at the patient's responses below, and state what the nurse might say next.

Patient's Response	*Nurse's Reply*

1. "It's just my state of mind, I guess. Would   YOUR ANSWER
you get me another glass of orange juice, please?"

CORRECT ANSWER

1. "Yes," or "I'm sorry, but you can't have extra juice on your diet."

Patient's Response	*Nurse's Reply*

2. "I'd just rather not talk about it."   **YOUR ANSWER**

CORRECT ANSWER

2. "All right, when will you be ready to take your bath?" (Or any response which changes the subject.)

C. RESPONDING TO SPECIFIC SITUATIONS

166

We have talked about instances when the nurse makes interpretations without sufficient information. There are two kinds of situations in which this is particularly likely to occur: when a patient resists treatment; and when he criticizes the hospital, the nurse herself, or some other member of the health team.

Because she feels defensive, she may act prematurely and try to force a treatment upon the patient or deny a criticism without finding out whether it is justified.

In the next few frames, we will present some ways in which the nurse might deal with these situations.

(Go on to the next frame.)

1. When the Patient is Critical

167

Patients occasionally criticize nurses, other members of the health team, or the services they are receiving. Sometimes, these criticisms are accurate appraisals and are clearly stated. At other times, the patient has a legitimate criticism, but his statement is too vague for the nurse to understand what it is. Finally, criticisms may reflect something other than dissatisfaction with the object of criticism. To clarify the meaning of the criticism, the nurse should elicit further description.

(Go on to the next frame.)

When a patient criticizes the hospital, the nurse should encourage him to give further information until she feels that his meaning is clear to her. Then she should check with him to find out if her interpretation is correct (i.e., she validates).

Patient's Thought	Patient's Comment	Nurse's Response	Patient's Reply	Nurse's Response
1. (This food is tasteless without salt.)	1. "I don't like the food. They didn't put salt on the tray."	1. "There isn't any salt on your tray, because you are on a low salt diet, but I will get you a salt substitute."	1. "Thank you."	1. "You're welcome."
2. (This food is tasteless without salt.)	2. "I don't like the food here."	2. "What's the matter?"	2. "They didn't put any salt on the tray and I'm used to eating my food with salt."	2. "There isn't any salt on your tray, because you are on a low salt diet. I will get you a salt substitute."
3. (I don't like the food or anything else about being here in the hospital.)	3. "I don't like the food here."	3. "What's the matter?"	3. "It doesn't taste good, but then I guess nothing would really taste good because I just don't like being here."	3. "Would you like to talk to me about it?"

168

169

When the patient criticizes impersonal aspects of hospitalization, the nurse may find it relatively easy to elicit information from the patient until she can identify the problem. When the object of the criticism is the physician or herself, however, she may be inclined to justify or defend the person or his actions. By so doing, she may be denying the patient the opportunity to fully express what he means. She may also cause the patient to see her as unsympathetic and may hinder the development of a therapeutic relationship in the long run. Below we have shown examples of patient's statements and nurse's responses which are ineffective.

1. Patient: "I don't want you to practice on me!"

   Student nurse: "But I know how to do it."

2. Patient   "The doctor comes in and out so fast that he doesn't take time to listen to my questions."

   Nurse: "He does the best that he can. You know he has so many patients to see."

(Go on to the next frame.)

170

Below are the patient's statements and the nurse's replies from the preceding frame. How would you feel if you were the patient in these situations, and the nurse made these replies to you?

1. Patient: "I don't want you to practice on me!"

   Student nurse: "But I know how to do it."

2. Patient: "The doctor comes in and out so fast that he doesn't take time to listen to my questions."

   Nurse: "He does the best that he can. You know he has so many patients to see."

YOUR ANSWER

CORRECT ANSWER

Specific feelings vary. You might feel angry because the nurse's replies sounded hostile, or you might feel guilty because she made you feel that your comment was unjustified.

You would probably feel that you had not obtained information that explained the situation to your satisfaction, i.e., what she has said has not assured you of her competency or the doctor's interest in your condition.

171

When the patient makes a vague statement or one which is subject to more than one interpretation, the nurse needs to find out exactly what the patient means before she can help him or take any definite action. Comments that are apparently criticisms of the hospital or its personnel may have multiple meanings. Below are the patient's comments from the preceding frame along with several different meanings they could have.

Patient's Comments	*Possible Meanings*
1. "I don't want you to practice on me!"	A. Nursing students are too inexperienced to know what they are doing. B. I feel like a guinea pig with medical students, interns, and nursing students working on me all the time. C. I didn't like the way you did the treatment for me the last time.
2. "The doctor comes in and out so fast that he doesn't take time to listen to my questions."	A. He doesn't answer my questions. B. He is so brusque that I hesitate to ask him any questions. C. I wish there were someone who *could* answer my questions. D. I just wish there were someone who would take the time to talk with me.

(Go on to the next frame.)

172

The method of eliciting further description may be used when patients make statements that are critical of hospital personnel. See the examples below.

Patient's Thought	Patient's Comment	Nurse's Response	Patient's Reply	Nurse's Response
1. (Nursing students are too inexperienced to know what they are doing.)	1. "I don't want you to practice on me!"	1. "Oh?"	1. "I think you nursing students are too inexperienced to know what you are doing."	1. "My instructor has watched me do it, and she thinks I do a good job. Would you like for her to be here with me while I do it?"
2. (I don't like the way you did the treatment for me the last time.)	2. "I don't want you to practice on me!"	2. "Oh?"	2. "You put the bandages on too loosely, and they fell off right away."	2. "I'll put them on tighter this time, and you tell me how you like it."
3. (He's always in such a hurry that I don't want to delay him by asking questions.)	3. "The doctor comes in and out so fast that he doesn't take time to listen to my questions."	3. "Tell me about that."	3. "He is always so rushed that I hesitate to ask him any questions."	3. "Perhaps you could tell him that you have several questions you wish to ask him, and want to know when he will have enough time to answer them."
4. (I wish there was someone who *could* answer my questions.)	4. "The doctor comes in and out so fast that he doesn't take time to listen to my questions."	4. "Tell me about that."	4. "Oh, I wish there were someone who *would* answer my questions."	4. "I'd be happy to talk with you about the questions you have and answer those that I can."

(Go on to the next frame.)

173

A patient statement has been given below.

What should the nurse's initial response be?

Patient: "I've been here in the hospital for two days, and no one has paid any attention to me."

YOUR ANSWER

CORRECT ANSWER

Correct responses include any of the following:

"Tell me about it." "What do you mean?" "What happened?"

174

Below are two possible replies that the patient might give to the nurse's request to go on. State a response that the nurse might make in each case.

1.   "You're the first nurse I've seen in two days, and I haven't had anybody to talk to."

YOUR ANSWER

CORRECT ANSWER

1.   "I'd be happy to sit down and talk with you. What would you like to talk about?"

2.   "I'd like to have a television set, but I don't know how to get one."

YOUR ANSWER

CORRECT ANSWER

2.   "I'll find out how to order it," or "I'll have the television man come around and see you." (Or equivalent responses.)

2. When the Patient Refuses a Treatment

175

We have shown you how the nurse responds to patients' criticisms. In the next few frames we will show how the nurse should respond when the patient refuses a treatment.

Following are three hypothetical situations in which the patient refuses to practice crutch walking. The physician wants her to practice before she leaves the hospital. In which of the three interactions has the nurse been most effective? What has she done that makes this the most effective?

Example I

Miss Jacobs:	"Mrs. Patterson, it's time for you to practice walking with your crutches again."
Mrs. Patterson:	"Oh, I don't want to do that now."
Miss Jacobs:	"The doctor says that you must practice enough to become proficient before you are discharged."
Mrs. Patterson:	"I understand that! But I just don't feel like doing it!"
Miss Jacobs:	"Well, I'll have to call your doctor and see what he wants you to do."
Mrs. Patterson:	"I guess you will, because I'm not going to do it!"

Example II

Miss Jacobs:	"Mrs. Patterson, it's time for you to practice walking with your crutches again."
Mrs. Patterson:	"Oh, I don't want to do that now."
Miss Jacobs:	"You don't?"
Mrs. Patterson:	"It hurts too much."
Miss Jacobs:	"It won't hurt very much, just a little, perhaps. You're not used to using those muscles and there will be a little strain."
Mrs. Patterson:	"But it *isn't* muscle soreness!"
Miss Jacobs:	"I'll get the crutches and you start. (Gets crutches) There. Would you please try it?"
Mrs. Patterson:	(Walking slowly) "Oh, it hurts so much."
Miss Jacobs:	"Hmmmm . . ."
Mrs. Patterson:	"I've been *trying* to tell you. They rub so much under my arms that it's terribly sore there!"
Miss Jacobs:	"Yes, I can see that now. Perhaps the hand grip is too low."

Example III

Miss Jacobs:	"Mrs. Patterson, it's time for you to practice walking with your crutches again."
Mrs. Patterson:	"Oh, I don't want to do that now."
Miss Jacobs:	"You don't?"
Mrs. Patterson:	"It hurts too much."
Miss Jacobs:	"Where does it hurt?"
Mrs. Patterson:	"The crutches rub so much under my arms."
Miss Jacobs:	"Let me see you stand with them. Yes, it looks as though the hand grip is too low. I'll set it higher and that should prevent it from rubbing."
Mrs. Patterson:	"All right."
Miss Jacobs:	(Adjusts the hand grip and watches Mrs. Patterson walk with the crutches.) "How does that feel?"
Mrs. Patterson:	"That's fine! It doesn't hurt now. Thank you."

YOUR ANSWER

CORRECT ANSWER

The nurse was most effective in *Example III.* By eliciting further description she was able to identify the reason for the patient's resistance and to take action which permitted the doctor's order to be carried out with the patient's consent. Note that in *Example II* Miss Jacobs began to seek further information but took action before she had sufficient information.

176

It is apparent that when the nurse comes to a premature conclusion about what the patient means or what problem a patient may be talking about, either her later communication with the patient and any action she may take are ineffective, or effective action is delayed.

(Go on to the next frame.)

177

After the nurse found out that Mrs. Patterson resisted using the crutches because it was painful, further exploration might have identified any of these sources of pain:

1. As given, the hand grip was placed too low.
2. Mrs. Patterson was using the crutches incorrectly.
3. The pain was engendered by muscle soreness resulting from an unmodifiable aspect of the treatment.

With this additional information, the nurse would take action. In the first case, raise the hand grip; in the second case, teach the patient the correct way to use the crutches; in the third case, offer the patient pain medication if it is permitted by the doctor's order and if it seems warranted.

When the patient refuses a treatment because it is painful, what more should the nurse find out before taking action? Why?

YOUR ANSWER

CORRECT ANSWER

She should find out the source of the pain. Her action will depend upon the source.

178

The patient may resist treatment because of pain. If the pain is due to some extrinsic factor, such as the patient performing the exercise incorrectly or pressure on a part, it may be alleviated by showing the patient how to perform the exercise correctly or relieving the pressure. If the pain is engendered by some intrinsic or unmodifiable part of the treatment, then pain medication may be used. It is important that the nurse find out the cause of the patient's pain, so that she does not give pain medication indiscriminately when an allowable modification of the treatment would suffice to relieve the pain.

(Go on to the next frame.)

179

Assuming that the doctor's orders permit giving pain medication, in which of the following instances would it be correct to offer it? Why?

1. Mrs. Lotti reports her bandage has been put on so tightly that her leg is painful.
2. Mrs. Charles says that she has been given injections in her left arm so frequently that the site is painful.
3. Mr. Hudson finds it very painful to rotate his wrist as ordered by the doctor. He is exercising correctly.

CORRECT ANSWER

Medication should be offered only to Mr. Hudson, because his pain is caused by an intrinsic aspect of the treatment. In the other cases wrapping the bandage less tightly and changing the site of injection treats the specific cause of pain.

180

Although the anticipation of pain is a frequent cause of resisting a treatment, resistance also occurs when the patient is not clear about its purpose or is doubtful about its effectiveness. When we discussed orienting the patient to an imposed task, we emphasized that the patient should be told its purpose. If the purpose is still not clear to the patient, he may ask the nurse for an explanation when the treatment is repeated. She should answer his question, since it is his right to know. To say something like, "It is ordered by your physician," is not responsive to the question. Furthermore, it is unnecessarily evasive. For these reasons, it is desirable to tell the patient the purpose of the treatment. Read the examples on this page and the following page as illustrations of appropriate responses.

Mr. O'Hara: "I just was operated on two days ago. Why must I get up and walk around? I just want to lie here and hurt!"

Miss Freeman: "The exercise will help your sore muscles to regain their tone, Mr. O'Hara. I can bring you some pain medication a few minutes before you start, so you won't feel so stiff and sore as you walk."

Mr. O'Hara: "Anything that will help will be fine. I'll do it because I want to get out of here, but I still won't like it."

(Go on to the next frame.)

181

Here is another example in which the nurse responds to the patient's refusal to do a treatment.

Miss Rosen: "Mrs. Andrews, it's time for you to do full range of motion on your leg."

Mrs. Andrews: "Oh, not today. I just don't want to do it."

Miss Rosen: "You don't?"

Mrs. Andrews: "No, I've been doing it for a week now, and I don't really think it's made any difference."

Miss Rosen: "Do you know what effect the exercise is supposed to have on your leg?"

Mrs. Andrews: "Yes, I guess it's supposed to loosen the muscles and help me move my leg around better."

Miss Rosen: "That's right. The only way we can see if the purpose of the exercise has been accomplished is to see you do it. Would you try it now while I watch?"

Mrs. Andrews: "Well, okay. (Hesitantly.) But just for a minute."

Miss Rosen: (Watches her.) "There has been some improvement."

Mrs. Andrews: "It doesn't look like much to me."

Miss Rosen: "Remember the first day, you could hardly bend your knee or lift your leg more than a couple of inches off the bed. Now, you can bend it almost to a forty-five degree angle, and you can lift your leg higher too."

Mrs. Andrews: "Well, that's right, but I've been doing these exercises for a week."

Miss Rosen: "Yes, but it does take a while to get your muscles back in shape when your leg has been immobilized for two months."

Mrs. Andrews: "I suppose you're right. I guess I'll just have to bear with it. (Resignedly.) I'll go ahead with the exercises, now."

(Go on to the next frame.)

182

Even when the nurse has found out why the patient has refused a treatment and has carried out what she believes to be appropriate action, the patient may still refuse to do the treatment. The nurse then informs the physician either verbally or by writing in the nursing notes on the patient's chart that the treatment was refused and the reason it was refused. She should try to find out the reason for the patient's resistance, so that the doctor can decide what should be done.

(Go on to the next frame.)

183

Mr. Hart has refused to continue the physical therapy treatments to his paralyzed right arm. Which of the two statements below is more useful to the physician?

1. Mr. Hart reports that the physical therapy exercises have not had any effect on his right arm and refuses to do them any more.

2. Mr. Hart refused to do the physical therapy exercises.

YOUR ANSWER

CORRECT ANSWER

Number one is better, because the physician has sufficient information for action without further discussion.

184

Mr. Clarke's physician has ordered him to cough three times a day. When you come to his room to help him cough, he says, "I'm not going to do it!"

What do you want to accomplish by your response?

YOUR ANSWER

CORRECT ANSWER

Find out the specific cause of his resistance and ultimately have him do the treatment.

185

What would you do in each of the following instances? Mr. Clarke further defines the problem by saying:

1. "My incision pulls apart when I cough."

YOUR ANSWER

CORRECT ANSWER

1. Offer to splint the incision with a towel, so that it won't feel like it's separating.

2. "When I cough my muscles hurt across my abdomen and chest, and even around to my back."

YOUR ANSWER

CORRECT ANSWER

2. Offer a pain medication.

3. "I don't understand why I have to do it."

YOUR ANSWER

CORRECT ANSWER

3. Explain the purpose which you have looked up in a medical text in terms he can understand.

4. "I don't need to cough any more, because I feel so much better."

YOUR ANSWER

CORRECT ANSWER

4. Report to the physician that the patient refused to cough because he feels so much better.

186

The following process is useful when the patient resists treatment.

1. The nurse elicits further description until the patient's meaning is clear.
2. She validates with the patient that she understands the problem as the patient sees it.
3. From the information provided, she infers what action should be taken.
4. She takes action.

(Go on to the next frame.)

BEHAVIORAL OBJECTIVES:

When the patient asks a question about his diagnosis or prognosis, for example, "Do I have diabetes?" or "I wonder about my condition." the student will first convey to the patient that such questions will be answered only by the physician. Then she gives the patient the opportunity to express his feelings if he wishes and finds out if there is any additional information that she should relay to the physician and/or other members of the health team. (Frames 187–205)

3. When the Patient Asks Questions about His Diagnosis or Prognosis

187

When the patient talks about his own diagnosis, prognosis, or the results of diagnostic tests, several things may be going on in his mind: he may be seeking to receive or confirm information; he may wish to express his feelings and sort out his thoughts about what is happening to him; or he may be trying to decide how to deal with what is happening to him.

(Go on to the next frame.)

188

Today, there is growing discussion among physicians about whether it is the right of all patients to be given complete information about their diagnoses and prognoses. Some physicians provide full diagnostic information, others do not. Still others decide what the patient should be told on the basis of the particular diagnosis and their judgment of the patient. In deciding how much information should be given to the patient, the physician utilizes data obtained from the patient and his family, from nurses and other members of the health team, but the final decision is his. The physician also decides when and how this information should be conveyed. Therefore, unless the patient's physician specifically asks the nurse to relay diagnostic information to the patient, the nurse should *not* do so.

(Go on to the next frame.)

189

Patients occasionally ask nurses for diagnostic information. Although nurses should not convey information, they must respond in some way to patients. We may consider some responses that the nurse might make and examine the probable effects of these responses in order to arrive at a type of response that *is* appropriate. Of primary concern is the interpretation that the patient is likely to draw from the nurse's response. For example, suppose that a patient asks, "Do I have diabetes?" and the nurse answers by saying, "I don't know." What are some possible interpretations that the patient might make? Is saying that she does not know an effective way for the nurse to respond to diagnostic questions? Why or why not?

YOUR ANSWER

CORRECT ANSWER

Some of the possible interpretations are:

1. Simply that the nurse does not know.

2. The nurse does not know. She should have the information, if she is competent. Therefore, she is not competent.

3. She doesn't know now, but she probably will know later on. I'll ask her again later on.

4. She is avoiding my question, because she knows I do have diabetes and is afraid that knowing about it will upset me.

The response "I don't know" is likely to be ineffective, because it may suggest information (correct or erroneous), reflect on the nurse's competence, and encourage the patient to ask the nurse for the same information again.

190

Consider the following situation. What possible interpretations might Mr. Morse be expected to make?

Mr. Morse has been in the hospital for three days for an appendectomy. Last night he had sharp pains in the chest, difficulty in breathing, and an erratic and rapid heart beat. Miss Flack enters his room and the following conversation occurs.

Mr. Morse: "I'm really concerned that I have heart trouble. Do I?"
Miss Flack: "Oh, no, Mr. Morse, don't worry about that."

YOUR ANSWER

CORRECT ANSWER

Possible interpretations:

1. I don't have heart trouble

2. I *know* I have heart trouble and so does Miss Flack. She just doesn't want me to know.

3. It's easy for *her* to say, "don't worry." She's not the one who is sick.

4. Is there something else I should be worrying about?

191

If the nurse denies that the patient's concerns are real, this could be interpreted either as an untruthful attempt to reassure him or as evidence that there is in fact no basis for concern. Suppose that a patient *does* in fact have a heart condition, but he believes the nurse's implication that he does not. What two undesirable effects may result, if the patient infers he does not have a heart condition?

YOUR ANSWER

CORRECT ANSWER

1. She has given him false reassurance. He will have to face the truth later on.

2. He may be less willing to follow medical and nursing requirements and restrictions.

192

If we go outside the hospital setting, we may examine the immediate and later effects of reassuring a person that his fears are unfounded. What would you expect the effects to be in the following cases?

Incident	*Question*	*Response by Friend*
Gail has twice received the lowest score in chemistry. She has studied for two hours but can't grasp the material.	"Do you think I'll get a passing grade in chemistry?"	Don't worry about that. Look how long you've studied. You'll do all right in the end.
Fran had been dating Gil regularly for the last two months. He has not called her in the last week.	"Gil seems to have stopped calling me. I don't think I'll be seeing him anymore."	Oh, I'm sure you will. There is probably some good reason why he hasn't called.

YOUR ANSWER

CORRECT ANSWER

Gail and Fran might think their friends just wanted to make them feel better, even though they didn't really mean what they said. If they believed what their friends said, it would only delay the disappointment that might occur later on. It also might prevent Gail and Fran from taking action to solve the problem.

193

The point is that it is not enough to avoid answering patients' questions about their diagnoses and prognoses by stating that you do not know or by saying not to worry. These answers might convey something more than the nurse intends. Remembering that it is the physician who must decide what the patient should be told about his own diagnosis, what should the nurse find out from the patient?

YOUR ANSWER

CORRECT ANSWER

She should find out what the physician has told the patient.

194

Mrs. Jacobs says to the nurse, "I wonder if I have diabetes."

As a start toward finding out information about Mrs. Jacobs' reasons for asking this question, the nurse should ask her what the doctor has told her about her diagnosis.

The following are examples of questions the nurse would ask the patient to gain this information.

1. "Have you talked with your doctor about your diagnosis?"
2. "What has the doctor told you about your illness?"

(Go on to the next frame.)

195

The nurse's response to diagnostic questions should be independent of information available to her, since it is not her role to convey information of this sort to patients. What would you say to the patient in each of the following instances? Quote yourself.

Patient's question: "They did a blood test on me today. Do I have anemia?"

Information Available to the Nurse	*Response*
1. Test is complete. Anemia is indicated.	1. **YOUR ANSWER**
2. Test is complete. Anemia is ruled out.	2. **YOUR ANSWER**
3. Test results are not known to the nurse.	3. **YOUR ANSWER**

CORRECT ANSWER

None of the answers should convey information about the test results.
"Has the doctor talked with you about the results of the test?"

196

Patients sometimes ask questions which bear on the probability of eventual recovery or the likely long range effects of their illnesses, that is, their questions concern their own prognosis. For example, the following questions might be directed to the nurse:

1. Will I ever get well?"
2. Do you think I'll ever be able to play tennis again?
3. Will this treatment be able to cure my illness?
4. Do you think I'll ever be able to work a full day again?

Questions of this sort have the same status as diagnostic questions. What should the nurse say first when patients ask questions about long term effects of their illnesses?

YOUR ANSWER

CORRECT ANSWER

Have you talked about _____ with your doctor?

197

Suppose that in response to the nurse's question, "have you talked with the doctor about your illness?" Mrs. Jacobs replies, "No, I haven't." Remembering that only physicians may convey diagnostic information to patients, what would you say next?

YOUR ANSWER

CORRECT ANSWER

The nurse should refer the patient to the physician, saying something like. "The doctor is the one who will tell you whether or not you have diabetes when he gets the results of your tests and examinations."

198

Once you have explained to the patient that only the physician may answer diagnostic questions, there are two other things that you should do:

1. Give the patient the opportunity to express his feelings if he wishes.
2. Find out if there is additional information that you should relay to the physician and/or other members of the health team.

(Go on to the next frame.)

199

What would you add to the final nurse response?

Mrs. Jacobs: "I wonder if I have diabetes."

Nurse: "Have you talked with your doctor about your diagnosis?"

Mrs. Jacobs: "No, I haven't."

Nurse: "The doctor is the one who will tell you whether or not you have diabetes when he gets the results of your tests and examinations."

YOUR ANSWER

CORRECT ANSWER

1. "What makes you think you have diabetes?" or
2. "Do you have some reason for suspecting that you have diabetes?" or
3. "Could you tell me more about your reasons for asking?"

200

The nurse should continue the conversation with Mrs. Jacobs and let her express whatever is on her mind. In the course of the conversation, the nurse may find out some information that she should convey to the physician. This can be done either verbally or in writing on the patient's record.

(Go on to the next frame.)

201

Even though the patient has talked with the physician about his diagnosis, he may bring it up again with the nurse. He may wish to seek more information, to express his feelings about his diagnosis, or to begin to deal with the implications of his illness.

(Go on to the next frame.)

202

Below are three possible replies that Mrs. Jacobs might make in response to the nurse's question, "Have you talked with the doctor about your illness?"

What would the nurse say and/or do in each case?

Mrs. Jacobs' Replies	*Nurse Responses*
1. "Yes, he said that I do have diabetes, but I thought people with that had to take shots and he didn't say anything about that!"	1.
2. "Yes! He said that I *do* have diabetes! (Disgustedly.) I suppose I'll be living like a hermit, since I can't go out eating and drinking with my friends like I used to!"	2.
3. "Yes. He said that I do have diabetes and I'm really depressed about it."	3.

YOUR ANSWER

CORRECT ANSWER

1. Refer Mrs. Jacobs to the physician. Even though this seems like a straight-forward information question, the nurse might add, "Is there anything else you wanted to talk about regarding this?"
2. "You sound upset about possible changes in your style of living."
3. "What specifically depresses you?"

203

When the nurse refers a patient to his physician for answers to diagnostic questions, she is following a principle that is consistent with her response to other kinds of questions. This principle is that the nurse provides the opportunity for the patient to set realistic expectations. In the examples below we have indicated a nurse's statement together with the expectation she is setting for the patient.

Nurse's Statement	*Expectation Set for the Patient*
1. "Good morning, Mr. Corwin, I am Miss Forest. I am going to give you your 10:00 A.M. medication."	1. Specifies and limits her role to administration of the medication.
2. "You may feel a momentary sting when I give you this injection."	2. Defines kind and duration of pain to be expected.
3. "I can understand that you are interested in Mr. Held, but information about each patient's illness is confidential. Have you had much pain in your leg this afternoon?"	3. States that the patient should not expect that confidential information about another patient will be revealed.
4. "Have you talked with your doctor about your diagnosis?" (Patient replies.) "I think you should talk with the doctor about the questions you have regarding your diagnosis.	4. Implies that the physician rather than the nurse is the person to whom diagnostic questions should be directed.

(Go on to the next frame.)

204

Generally, when the nurse gives the patient the opportunity to set realistic expectations, he will follow her lead. For example, when the nurse indicates that the physician is the person who answers questions about diagnoses, then the patient does not pursue diagnostic questions with her. However, should the patient continue to ask questions about his diagnosis, what should the nurse say to the patient?

YOUR ANSWER

CORRECT ANSWER

Examples are:

"I can't answer that; the doctor is the person who should answer this kind of question."

"You should ask the doctor this question, since as a nurse I'm not permitted to answer it."

(Or any answer where the nurse clearly states that answering questions about the patient's diagnosis is the function of the physician and not of the nurse.)

205

As you finish making Mrs. Fulton's bed, she has a coughing spell. After it is over she says, "This isn't the way my asthma usually affects me. Do you think that I have pneumonia?"

1. What three things do you want to accomplish in your response?
2. Write down your response as you would make it to Mrs. Fulton.

YOUR ANSWER

CORRECT ANSWER

1.　a.　Tell Mrs. Fulton that it is the doctor, rather than the nurse, who answers diagnostic questions.
　　b.　Get information to convey to the doctor concerning the reasons for her suspicions.
　　c.　Let Mrs. Fulton express her feelings and/or begin to deal with any implications of her illness.

2.　"Mrs. Fulton, only the physician will be able to tell you if you have pneumonia. Has he talked with you about this or what has led you to suspect that you might have pneumonia?"

D. CREATING AN ATMOSPHERE WHERE COMMUNICATION IS MOST LIKELY TO OCCUR

BEHAVIORAL OBJECTIVES:

When examples of the following nurse responses occur in an interaction, the student identifies them as useful or not useful, and if not useful, states an appropriate alternative response. (Frames 206–241)

Not Useful
　　1.　Imposing value judgments
　　2.　Using withdrawal techniques
　　　　a.　Withdrawing from the situation physically
　　　　b.　Changing the subject, either entirely, or by responding to parts of the patient's statements that are remote from the problem he is discussing.
　　　　c.　Becoming very involved in performing physical care.
　　　　d.　Focusing on facts rather than feelings.
　　　　e.　Reassuring the patient without factual basis.

Useful
　　1.　Responding to feeling
　　2.　Clarifying ambiguities
　　3.　Using silence
　　4.　Validating impressions with the patient
　　5.　Providing information

206

As you have noted, throughout the interactions presented thus far in the program, the nurse has had an effect upon the patient. Effective interactions with the patient enable him to better express and understand his own feelings, adjust to his illness, and move toward his own level of optimum health.

One of the most important things you will learn in your clinical experience is the effects that you have upon your patients. When the effects are other than you would like you should be able to discover why and begin to change your behavior.

207

A verbatim (or process recording) is a written record of the verbal and non-verbal exchanges between the nurse and the patient during an interaction. This information can either be recorded via tape, while the interaction is in progress, or written down by the student, as soon after the interaction as possible.

When the student is able to look more closely at what she and the patient have said to each other and how they have reacted to each other, she develops an increased awareness of her non-verbal and verbal behavior patterns and their effect. This enables her to learn more about herself and her behavior in certain situations. It also helps her to learn these same things about the patient to his benefit in receiving better and more individualized nursing care.

Below is a sample of what kind of information should be included in a verbatim, and one way to set it up.

SAMPLE VERBATIM

Data:
Students' name
Patients' initials
Background information
    Brief medical history, including diagnosis
    Family data

Setting the scene of the interaction

Nurse	*Patient*	*Analysis*
1. What the nurse said, including voice tone.	1. What the patient said, including voice tone.	1. Purpose of nurse's response.
2. The nurse's non-verbal behavior	2. The patient's non-verbal behavior	a. Does it encourage the patient to express what is on his mind?
a. What she is doing	a. Body posture	b. Does it provide information to the patient when he needs it?
b. Facial expressions	b. Facial expressions	2. How her response affects the patient's behavior.
c. Mannerisms	c. Mannerisms	3. Is nurse's response useful or not useful? If not useful, what response would be better?
3. Nurse's feelings		

(Go on to the next frame.)

208

Here is an example taken from a verbatim:

Patient:　Mrs. M.　Age 83
Medical History:　Diabetic. Admitted to hospital with ulcer on right lower leg 4 days ago. Skin graft from right thigh to right lower leg at ulcer site.
Family Data:　Lives alone in old house in Chelsea.

This is a portion of the conversation which occurred after most of the morning care had been completed.

Nurse	Patient	Analysis
How do you feel now, Mrs. M.?	Oh, I haven't the strength of a cat! I'm so tired. You know there seems to be nothing but sickness and trouble for a body nowdays. I have a friend in the hospital now.	Earlier she had complained of being uncomfortable because of her dirty bed. I wanted to see if morning care had been helpful.
You do?	Yes, she's in Detroit. She's been there for quite a while. (Slight pause.) (She looked as though she was going to say something else.) You know my daughter was in the hospital.	I wanted to find out more about this friend and her hospitalization and if the patient was relating the friend's hospitalization to her own.
Oh?	She had kidney trouble and she died. She waved goodbye to one of my other daughters when she went to the hospital and the next morning they called her at six o'clock and she was dead. Can you imagine that? She was only 57, and she died. I was afraid the same thing was going to happen to me before I had this leg fixed here. (She points to right leg.)	Mrs. M. had been very anxious when I had cared for her the previous week (before her operation) and I wanted to find out just what her hospitalization meant to her. I knew that a daughter had died recently but I did not know under what circumstances. I thought perhaps she was relating her daughter's hospitalization to her own and thus encouraged her to tell more about her daughter.
You were afraid you might die?	Yes, but the operation wasn't bad.	I wanted to make sure I understood what the patient had said.
You know that everyone who has kidney disease doesn't die and everyone who comes to the hospital certainly doesn't die.	Oh yes, but it still made me worry.	I wanted her to realize that hospitalization need not mean death. However, my statement took the focus away from her particular problem and generalized too much. I might better have said, "Tell me about the operation."
How do you think your leg is doing now?	Oh, I don't know. Everyone says it's coming along fine, but I don't know.	I wondered if the patient was still worrying about dying and wanted to find out what she thought of her present condition.

Nurse	*Patient*	*Analysis*
You don't know?	(No reply)	By her tone of voice and what she had said, it seemed as though there were something she was holding back, and I wished to find out what she did mean.
I don't think I understand what you mean.	Well, I don't think it's going to get better. Everyone says it's getting better but I don't think so.	
What makes you say that?	Well, I've been here for two weeks on Tuesday and that's quite a while.	I wished to find the reason for the patient's statement.
Yes, but your leg does look good and it does take time for it to heal and it seems as though you're stronger than you were last week.	Yes, but I don't know if I'll get better or not. I'm first going to trust in the Almighty and hope that He'll let me get better because I want to get out of here.	From my knowledge of this patient, it seemed as though she had a good chance for recovery. She was despondent about being in bed for so long and I wanted her to see the "brighter" side of the situation too. However, in Mrs. M's reply, I felt she revealed how she intended to face the situation. She was not overly confident but she still had hope.
Have you thought about what you'll do right after you get out of the hospital?	Yes, I'm going to stay with my daughter for a while after I get out. Then I think I'll get a day bed and have someone come in and care for me.	I knew that the patient lived alone and I thought that she would probably need some help right after leaving the hospital.
You used to live alone, didn't you, Mrs. M.?	Yes, I even did my own washing but I had my daughter come over and hang it up.	In the patient's statement, I could again see a suggestion that she thought she would never get well again, at least not completely well. I didn't want Mrs. M. to resign herself to spending the rest of her life in bed.
Were you able to get around until you injured your leg?	Oh, yes.	
But you seem to think you won't get around anymore. Is that right?	I guess so. I don't know about this leg.	I was trying to help the patient, as well as myself, see what her feelings were.

Nurse	*Patient*	*Analysis*
Well, there is certainly a chance that you'll be up again.	Oh, I hope so, I hope so. I'll just trust in the Almighty.	I was again trying to reassure the patient that there was a chance for recovery which she had apparently thought improbable as revealed by her previous statements. She keeps returning to the uncertainty about her leg healing. And I keep reassuring her—which doesn't help her, as I see in retrospect. Perhaps I could have asked her what her doctor had said about how her leg was coming.
(Pause) I see you have a folder here from the Chapel.	A folder? (She seemed somewhat surprised.)	Her reference to God made me wonder if she might want to see the Chaplain, and thus I wished to investigate this area.
(I showed her the folder that had been lying on her table.)	Oh, yes, The Chaplain sees me and another lady in here. He's such a jolly character.	
Does he come often?	Oh, yes! He comes every morning—after Mass. I guess it's good to see him.	
I imagine you look forward to seeing him.	Yes, he's so nice.	This statement was not really necessary and had no special purpose.

(Go on to the next frame.)

209

Here are three interactions. In each one, the patient begins by making the same comment, yet his interaction with the nurse continues differently in each example. What accounts for this difference?

Example I.
Mr. Goble: "Nobody cares about me!"
Miss Wilder: "All of us here in the hospital are interested in you, Mr. Goble."
Mr. Goble: "That's what all the nurses say!"

Example II.
Mr. Goble: "Nobody cares about me!"
Miss Wilder: "Oh, but your family has visited you several times since you've been here, Mr. Goble!"
Mr. Goble: "That isn't what I meant! You just don't understand, do you?"

Example III.
Mr. Goble: "Nobody cares about me!"
Miss Wilder: "Tell me what you mean, Mr. Goble."
Mr. Goble: "I guess what I mean is that, even though I know that my family cares about me, and you nurses and doctors too, I am still the one who has to face this illness, and I am going through it by myself. I just feel lonely at times."

CORRECT ANSWER

The differences in the nurse's behavior:
In the first two examples, she denies the validity of this feelings.
In the last example, she encourages him to clarify what he means.

210

As you observe your behavior, deliberately trying to find out how what you are contributes to your relationships with patients, you will begin to find out answers to the following questions.

1. What do I do when patients are angry? Critical? Depressed? Anxious?
2. How do I respond when patients want to discuss their feelings about impending death?
3. What do I do when I feel inadequate to handle a situation?
4. What ways do I use to encourage patients to describe their feelings?

As you find out the answers to these questions, you will discover aspects of your behavior that you wish to change, and will begin to change them.

(Go on to the next frame.)

211

When you begin looking at your own behavior, you will probably see yourself moving through three levels. At first, you may not know what would be the best thing to say in a given situation, even looking back upon it in retrospect. As you progress, you will know what should have been said, although you may not have been able to say it at the time. Finally, you will more consistently say the correct thing at the appropriate time.

In the following examples you will see how the same student might respond to the same situation as her skills develop.

Level I

Nurse	Patient	Analysis
(While giving bed bath) Is your wife coming in to see you this morning?	(Irritably) She's staying here.	
Oh I see.	She just went to get some breakfast.	
Then I guess she'll be back soon.	I'm already too much of a burden on her now.	
Oh, I'm sure you're not.	Could you get some hotter water? (1)	(1) I felt that he didn't want to talk about his wife anymore so he changed the subject.
Of course, I'll be right back.		

Level II

Nurse	*Patient*	*Analysis*
(While giving bed bath) Is your wife coming in to see you this morning?	(Irritably) She's staying here.	
Oh, I see.	She just went to get some breakfast.	
Then I guess she'll be back soon.	I'm already too much of a burden on her now.	
Oh, I'm sure you're not. (1)	Could you get some hotter water?	(1) This was a *very* bad thing to say for it cut the patient off right away and showed him that I didn't understand and didn't want to talk about his problem with him. I realized what I had done as soon as I said it, but that was too late. I think it all gets back to my being nervous about the patient's condition, so that I wasn't ready for a deep discussion of his problems. Perhaps if I had been in a different emotional state I could have said, "Tell me about your feelings of being a burden."
Of course, I'll be right back.		

Level III

Nurse	*Patient*	*Analysis*
(While giving bed bath) Is your wife coming in to see you this morning?	(Irritably) She's staying here.	
Oh, I see.	She just went to get some breakfast.	
Then I guess she'll be back soon.	I'm already too much of a burden on her now.	
Tell me about your feelings of being a burden. (1)	She has run and fetched for me for so many months, I feel as though she needs a rest.	(1) I used a general statement here to allow the patient to describe his feelings as fully as he cared to.
(Nods) (2)	She hasn't been well either. She had a virus just after I came here, etc.	(2) My non-verbal response also encouraged him to continue.

(Go on to the next frame.)

212

The student learns that if you offer a choice to the patient when there can be no choice it is a frustrating experience for both. Moreover, the patient may not receive something that he needs.

Look at the following example.

Nurse	*Patient*	*Analysis*
Would you like me to rub your lower back now? You could turn to the right like you did when I helped you wash your back and I will put pillows here and here (pointing) so you won't have to hold yourself up.	Not right now. I am too tired. That pill made me sleepy.	This situation arose as a result of my giving the patient a choice when there wasn't any, because she needed good skin care. There wasn't even much of a choice as to time because we had saved the backrub until last so she could rest up. I allowed her to form expectations which weren't in keeping with the situation by giving her a choice. This experience has certainly been a good example of why one doesn't offer the patient a choice when he doesn't have one. It was frustrating for both me and the patient to have to hassle over this. In the future, I'll sure try to avoid offering a choice when there isn't any.
It would be a good idea for me to do it thoroughly to keep your skin from getting sore again.	No, I am too tired. (Patient turns head and shuts eyes, as if going to sleep.)	

I'll give you a few minutes to rest and then I'll be back. (I left to talk with my instructor.)

More generally, when a student analyzes her interaction with a patient and sees instances where she could have been more effective, what should happen the next time she finds herself in a similar situation?

YOUR ANSWER

CORRECT ANSWER

Her behavior should change and she should improve.

213

Read the following interactions and the analyses. (1) In each case state whether or not the nurse's last response was useful and write a comment she would make in the analysis column. (2) If she should have responded differently, suggest a substitute.

Interaction I

Nurse: Miss Chivera	*Patient: Mrs. Kamson*	*Analysis*
Have you been weak like this for a long time?	I have multiple sclerosis. Do you know what that is?	
I remember studying about it in anatomy, but I don't remember a lot about it right now.	I have had this for 4½ years now. I suppose I could have some disease that is worse though.	
Yes, that's true. I think that is a good attitude to have.	Yes, I suppose so. I shouldn't spend my time worrying about it, should I?	

Interaction II

Nurse: Miss Ficas	Patient: Mr. Zilsky	*Analysis*
(While putting a soak on his leg.)	Probably just about the time you get that thing on, the "big boss" will come and take it all off.	
Is he coming this morning?	No, he's in California now. He's one of those big "Teaching Doctors," hasn't got time for his patients. In fact, that's why they put all these restrictions on me. It will look bad for the "Chief Surgeon" if I don't get well.	
You don't like him?	No, it's not that. He's just too busy teaching. If I don't get well, it won't look good for him. That's all it is, just a bunch of politics. That's all medicine is!	
Well, I don't know about that, but I can understand your frustration at being in the hospital again so soon this way.	Yeh, I don't like being here one bit!	

YOUR ANSWER

CORRECT ANSWER

1. In *Interaction I,* Miss Chivera's last response was not useful.
Her analysis might have been—"Here I made a judgement which I shouldn't have done. I cut her off from any expression of feelings she might have cared to make by praising her for finding the best in her situation."
In *Interaction II,* Miss Ficas' last response was useful.
Her analysis might have been— "I'm trying to maintain a non-judgmental attitude, but finding it hard to do. I want to keep from making judgmental statements in order to encourage him to express his feelings about his own hospitalization. This worked, because he finally started to talk about how he felt.

2. Both nurses recognized that a moralistic or judgmental response would not encourage the patient to express himself. Miss Chivera only recognized this in retrospect. She might have said instead, "Four and ½ years is a long time to be ill." or "That's true, but you do have this one."

214

Two interactions follow
1. What were both students trying to accomplish at the beginning?
2. What did the students do when they began to achieve their beginning goals?
3. What motivated them to do this?
4. Looking at the analyses, at which level was each student?

Interaction I

Nurse: Miss Werly	*Patient: Mr. T.*	*Analysis*
	(Has been eating half a popsicle while conversing with Miss Werly about a variety of things. Now he begins to smoke) I guess I won't be smoking much longer though I really don't see what difference it would make.	
What do you mean? (1)	I already have cancer. I don't have to worry about smoking. I'd suspected it for quite awhile but they didn't tell me for sure until last night. (He was fidgeting with his cigarette in the ashtray. (2)	(1) Mr. T. continues to express his feelings. The question I asked next may have been too obvious. It was meant to help the patient recapitulate his thoughts and thereby understand himself better.
What are your feelings this morning? (3)		(2) Mr. T. was a little hesitant at first. After the first sentence, he looked up as if to see if he had shocked me.
	I feel better this morning. They gave me a shot to calm me. I'd really like to go home. I figure when it gets near the end I'll go home to stay. (Pointing to the IV's) They can shove these things in me at home as well as in here. The Doctors only gave me four to six months to live. But they're going to try something that may give me a couple of years. I'm not making any plans for the future, though, because I don't know if I'll be around. I'll let my wife handle that.	(3) Mr. T. had verbalized some of his feeling, which may have been the first time. I wanted him to do this so that he might view his problem more realistically and possibly begin to accept it.
(There is a pause) (4)	(Looks at nurse and then looks away)	(4) I failed to think of any other question I could ask.
(I felt that it was a little cool so I got up to shut the window) (5)	I think I'd like the other half of that popsicle. (5)	(5) Mr. T. saw this as an opportunity to stop talking about himself. He may have wanted to be left alone for a little while.
Certainly, I'll be right back.		

Interaction II

Nurse: Miss Adams	*Patient: Mr. H.*	*Analysis*
(I entered the unit and introduced myself.)	Oh, you're my helper this morning, huh?	
(I nodded and inquired as to how he was feeling.)	I have been here a little longer than I expected. I thought at first it would be only about three weeks. This has upset my plans a little. . . . Let's see . . . it's been five weeks now. (6)	(6) Mr. H. made this observation almost immediately. Superficially, he seems to have worked through some feelings about his illness, realizing that it upset his plans; but I think now there was a deeper fear and he needed to talk about it.
How much longer do you expect to be here? (7)	They don't say. I thought my nerves would give out before now, but they seem to have held up pretty well. (His hands were trembling and his arm muscles twitched.)	(7) I really did not give him this opportunity. Perhaps I could have said, "Yes, I can see how this would upset one's plans" and then perhaps asked the question, It might have helped the patient to clarify his feelings.
(I remained silent and proceeded with his morning care.) (8)		(8) I could have asked for clarification of his response, and to his comment about his nerves, I could have responded, "You feel that you have withstood the strain of your illness quite well." Instead of this, I withdrew from the situation, a relief behavior to the anxiety I was experiencing in myself. I don't know if the patient knew that he had cancer. I think perhaps this may have been the underlying cause of his anxiety. I didn't realize this at the time.

YOUR ANSWER

CORRECT ANSWER

1. Trying to encourage the patient to express his feelings.
2. They felt inadequate to deal with what they had elicited and they withdrew.

3. They were uncomfortable in the situation and wanted to reduce their own anxiety or to remove themselves from a situation with which they felt unable to cope.

4. Miss Werly is at Level I
   Miss Adams is at Level II

215

Sometimes, when the nurse is in a situation with which she cannot cope, or that makes her anxious, she does things that help her to get out of the situation or lessen her own anxiety.

These are such actions as:

1. Withdrawing from the situation physicially.
2. Changing the subject either entirely or by responding to parts of the patient's statements that are remote from the problem he is discussing.
3. Becoming very involved in performing physical care.
4. Focusing repeatedly on the facts that the patient is discussing rather than the feelings.
5. Reassuring the patient without factual basis.

All the ways of coping listed above involve removing herself in some way from the patient and his problem or making the problem seem more remote. Although she is doing this to help herself cope, the patient is not likely to be hurt. He will undoubtedly try to find someone else to whom he can express himself.

We believe that the nurse cannot indefinitely rely on these actions because they hinder her own growth and her ability to make it easier for the patient to state what is on his mind. As long as she is using these avoidance techniques she is not fulfilling one of the most important functions of the nurse: to help the patient attain his own level of optimum health.

Thus, she needs to begin to know what situations provoke her use of them, and take steps to examine her own feelings so that she is less anxious and better able to cope.

(Go on to the next frame.)

216

There is one way you can respond when you are anxious and unable to cope which requires rather little on your part and yet does not remove you from the patient. Rather than using these avoidance techniques, you can remain with the patient and show either non-verbally or verbally your interest in what he is saying. That is, you nod, murmur "um-hum" and look with interest at the patient. Very often this may serve to let him state what is on his mind.

Following is an example of a beginning nursing student who did just this.

Date:
Student:
Patient: Mr. J. L.
Background: 49 years old.
　　　　　　 Diagnosis—Leukemia.
　　　　　　 Has been in the hospital for 3 weeks.
　　　　　　 Married, has 2 grown children—works as a piano tuner.

Nurse:	Patient:	Analysis
(It was about 9:15 and the patient had just finished breakfast. I stopped by his unit to see if he was ready to take his bath.) Are you about ready for your bath, Mr. L.?	Yes, I can't take a hot shower anymore—the doctors are afraid the steam and heat will make me faint.	I wanted to see if the patient was ready to bathe. Because there was not a great deal that I would be doing, I didn't want to rush into his care if he would rather wait for a little while.

Nurse	Patient	Analysis
Yes, you understand that they want you to take a sponge bath rather than a shower?	Yes, I know.	I wanted to validate with the patient that he understood that the doctor's orders prohibited all showers both hot and cold—and allowed him to take only a sponge bath.
	(Pause) You know, I think this 6 MP they are giving me must be stronger than _____ (naming a drug with which I was not familiar)	
Do you?		Because I was not familiar with the particular drug he mentioned I should have elicited further information about it. I probably should have said something like: "I don't believe I'm familiar with _____, can you tell me about it?" Had I done this I might possibly have learned why he was comparing the two. As it turned out, his next comment provided me with some of the information I should have tried to uncover.
	Yes, I took _____ at the beginning of my illness, but now they have me on 6 MP. I think they have something to do with depressing the bone marrow. Only I think 6 MP is stronger. I suppose when this drug loses its effect they will give me one that is stronger still.	
Possibly.		I really had no ideas what to say here. Since I didn't know what type of treatment his doctors had planned for him I was afraid of giving him false information, so I selected a noncommital answer. Perhaps it would have been better had I simply said: "I don't know."
	I've often wondered what happens when all the bone marrow is destroyed. But I suppose they never have found out—nobody who has what I have is ever around after two years, so I guess they don't have time to find out.	

Nurse	*Patient*	*Analysis*
		I was left completely speechless, not knowing quite how I should react. I wasn't sure that Mr. L. had been told that he had leukemia. I had assumed he had from his conversation with Mr. R. but because I wasn't certain about this point I was afraid to say anything that might give validity to any suspicions he might have were he merely "fishing." As a result I didn't say anything. Perhaps I should have elicited further information and attempted to discover the source of his information. But I didn't feel that I could do this.
	(Pause) Of course, I've always said that I'm going to beat this thing.	
(Nodding yes and softly murmuring "uh-huh")		Here again I was at a loss for words. My nodding and "uh-huh" were intended to mean "I understand—tell me more" and I think the patient understood what I meant. I was unable to say anymore—everything I considered saying sounded awkward, and this was all I could get out.
	They are always doing research and you never know when they are going to come up with something that will be a cure. Dr. Simpson—he's related to the Simpson for whom the institute was named—told me that they don't really look for a cure in the near future, but he said that there was always the possibility.	
(Nodding yes and softly murmuring "uh-huh")		I wanted so very much to tell him that I was sure they would discover a cure and everything would be all right. But I realized that this would be false reassurance and would do more harm than good. The temptation was great, but I couldn't tell him everything would be all right when both of us knew it wouldn't. I know that I should

Nurse	*Patient*	*Analysis*

Analysis (right column top): have responded to him in a more suitable manner than I did. Perhaps I could have said something like "Yes, they might develop a cure, but, as you say, no one really knows."

Patient: You never can tell. But still, I have a family to think about. There are a lot of things I need to take care of. I'm glad the kids are older. You know I told you, my daughter is an RN and my son is a freshmen in collge.

Nurse: Yes, I remember.

Analysis: The patient was obviously quite worried about his family and what would happen to them. Perhaps I could have helped verbalize some of his anxiety had I said something like: "You are worried about your family" Although my reply did not cut him off I certainly missed a very important cue.

Patient: (Pause) It's an old cliché, but it's true—there are times when you just can't fight city hall. And I guess this is one of those times. I don't want to just give up, I'm going to give it all I've got, but sometimes that isn't enough. I'll just have to wait and see—I'm afraid there isn't much else I can do. Well, do you think you can get me some clean pajamas? I'll wash up in the bathroom while you make my bed. (Pause during which the patient stared at the bed. Then he sighed and looked up at me and smiled.)

Nurse: Certainly. And this time I'll promise to find you some that fit.

Analysis: The patient, himself, terminated the conversation. Apparently he had said what was on his mind and was ready to move on to other things. Two weeks before, when I had this same patient I had gotten him a pair of pajamas that were so small that he could hardly get them buttoned. I guess I was relieved when the conversation moved to something else and I

Nurse	*Patient*	*Analysis*

Analysis:

needed some sort of release from the tension that I had built up during the conversation and I started teasing him about lighter matters. He must have sensed this because his next remark reflected this same lightness. I hope that I didn't convey the impression that I found what he had said to be unacceptable because I didn't at all. I had the feeling that he, himself, was ready for a change of mood too.

Patient:

(Smiling) I'll bet you can't—they only have them in two sizes here; too small and too large.

Too large.

Nurse:

Well, in that case, which would you rather have—too large or too small?

Well, I'll see what I can do. I'll be right back.

Analysis:

I can see from this verbatim that I didn't handle the conversation very well. It's easy to see what I should have said in some of these places, but it is much more difficult to actually say them. I was very uneasy during the conversation, but I tried to hide it as much as I could. I have so many unresolved questions about death, myself, that I felt very incompetent about talking with someone who is facing the ordeal himself. I have never lost anyone close to me so I can't honestly say that I felt the full impact of what he was saying. My uneasiness prevented me from making many of the responses that I should have made. I just didn't know what to say to him. All I could do was to listen and hope that by just being there I could help him. I certainly didn't give him any support in any other way.

I think doing this verbatim has really helped me to recognize some of my own feelings that I had never analyzed before. I hope that when this situation arises again I will know where

Nurse	*Patient*	*Analysis*
		my own difficulties lie, be more able to focus on the needs of the patient and to give him more assurance.

What good things came out of the fact that the student remained with the patient?

YOUR ANSWER

CORRECT ANSWER

1. The patient talked.
2. The student was able, in retrospect, to see where she might have interjected encouraging responses.
3. The student became aware of some of her own feelings that she felt needed further examination.
4. She was able to see herself as coping with a situation that she knew was difficult.

217

In some of the frames that follow, we will be asking you to decide whether or not a nurse's specific response is useful.

If a response is useful, you should be able to answer "Yes." to the following questions: Is it responsive to what the patient has said? And, if information is required, does the response provide it? Does it encourage the patient to express himself as opposed to cutting him off prematurely?

In making your judgment about the usefulness of the nurse's response, look not only at how well it relates to what the patient said before but look at the patient's response to it.

(Go on to the next frame.)

218

On the same day, Mr. Wilson brought up the same subject to two different nurses, Miss Rogers and Miss Baker. We want to contrast these two interactions because we think that they illustrate several of the points we have discussed in the book.

Mr. Wilson is a 51 year old car salesman who has been bothered in recent years by a chronic urinary tract infection. One week ago he had an operation to repair a urethral stricture. His post-operative course has been normal and he will be able to be discharged from the hospital in approximately one more week. Four days ago, Mr. Wilson's father died in a distant city. The funeral was yesterday. Read the interaction between Mr. Wilson and Miss Rogers and then answer the following questions.

1. Look specifically at Miss Rogers' comments, numbered 1 through 3. For each one, state:
    a. Is the response useful?
    b. Why the response is not useful (where applicable).
    c. An alternative response, if the original response was not useful.
2. What does Miss Rogers do that suggests that she is trying to avoid dealing with Mr. Wilson's feelings about his father's death?

Interaction I: Mr. Wilson and Miss Rogers

Miss Rogers	*Mr. Wilson*	*Analysis*
Well, how was your breakfast? You know, Mr. Wilson, it's very important to eat all of your food so that you gain your strength back quickly. (1)	Just so-so. I didn't eat it all.	I noticed that he left much of his breakfast on his plate and I took this opportunity to remind him how important it is for an ill person to eat.
	(Silence. Stares at nurse briefly.)	He looked so strained after I made my comment that I thought perhaps I should have found out why he didn't eat all of his breakfast.
Mr. Wilson, have you had your bath yet? (2)	No, I am going to take a shower, shave, and fix my teeth now.	This question was just to obtain necessary information.
All right. I will get you some clean towels and pajamas.		This was to confirm his judgment and to show him I would abide by his decisions. I wanted to tell him that I was going to get his pajamas.
(Returned with pajamas.) Here you are.	(He took the pajamas and handed me a memorial card from a funeral.) This is from my father's funeral. He died a few days ago and the funeral was yesterday.	I felt very uneasy at this point. It is always a very difficult situation when someone talks about a recently deceased relative. I didn't want to merely say "I'm sorry," because it sounds rather trite and I did want to learn more about the situation without creating more anxiety than was present, so I used a reflective question.
He died a few days ago?	Yes, he was 89 years old when he died. He hadn't been sick a day in his life. He was very active right up to the end. He had a good life. (Pause.)	The question did evoke more information. I knew he wanted to talk about it because he introduced the subject and I knew he wanted to terminate it because he closed the subject. From his facial expressions and actions, I assumed that he was very well adjusted to the loss and when he chose to close the subject, I did not press the issue and create more anxiety than was already present.
I will make your bed while you take your shower. (3)	(Pause.) Okay. I'll go ahead now and take my shower.	

YOUR ANSWER

1.

1. a.

    b.

    c.

2. a.

    b.

    c.

3. a.

    b.

    c.

2.

CORRECT ANSWER

1.
1. a. The response is not useful.
    b. Miss Rogers didn't find out the reason Mr. Wilson was not eating and she moralized to him.
    c. "I noticed that you didn't eat it all."
2. a. The response is not useful.
    b. Mr. Wilson's silence gave a clue that perhaps he had reason for not eating but Miss Rogers avoided following it up.
    c. Same as 1.c. or "You're rather quiet. Is there something bothering you?"
3. a. The response is not useful.
    b. Miss Rogers changes the subject without any indication from Mr. Wilson that he has finished the topic. The fact that he pauses after Miss Rogers' comment and doesn't continue his topic gives a clue that her comment was not useful.
    c. "His death was quite unexpected, then."
2. a. Miss Rogers concentrates on physical activities (making the bed and taking a shower) which make it unnecessary for her to have to deal with Mr. Wilson's feelings.
    b. She assumed, without adequate basis, that the patient wanted to terminate talking about his father. Her analysis suggests that her own anxiety led her to make this assumption.

The interaction between Miss Rogers and Mr. Wilson has been a classic example of the nurse avoiding the patient's expression of feelings because she herself felt unable to cope with them. In the contrasting example below, Miss Baker successfully found out what Mr. Wilson was feeling and encouraged him to express himself.

Read the interaction between Miss Baker and Mr. Wilson and then answer the following questions.

3. Note three things that helped Miss Baker identify what Mr. Wilson was feeling.

4. What three things did Miss Baker do to help Mr. Wilson express his feelings?

Interaction II: Mr. Wilson and Miss Baker

Miss Baker	*Mr. Wilson*	*Analysis*
	Hello, Miss Baker. How are you feeling?	
Very well, Mr. Wilson.	I once sold a car to a man named Baker. Let's see, that was way back in '67. He was from Muskegon. Any relation?	
No, I don't think so. Mr. Wilson, it amazes me how you remember names.	Well, that's part of my business, you know. I'm a salesman and I've found it's really important to remember details about people—salesmanship. I've sort of developed systems of associating items, etc.	
(I made no specific verbal response to his conversation, but I was looking at him while he was talking)	(We begin walking back to his bedside as he continued to describe his work.)	
	(When we reach his bedside, he begins to place the articles he was carrying on the bedside stand. He picks up a card from the stand and hands it to Miss Baker) This is the memorial card from my father's funeral.	
Your father was buried yesterday? (We were still standing at the bedside.)	Yes. He died rather suddenly last Saturday.	I notice that the date of the service was yesterday. I was carefully observing Mr. Wilson's face to notice any behavior that would indicate his feelings. I saw no change of expression and there was nothing indicative in his voice.
Oh? (Sitting down in chair.)	(Sat on edge of bed.) He was 89—hadn't been sick at all, and he was always extremely active for his age. I think he had a good life. (Short pause. Still no further clues from face or voice.)	
You weren't able to go to the funeral.	No, but my sister flew here from Florida and she gave me a complete report. Evidently it was a very nice service. (Pause) I was quite worried about the arrangements. (Voice broke, eyes appeared watery.)	

Miss Baker	*Mr. Wilson*	*Analysis*
Tell me more about this, Mr. Wilson.	Well, since I was here, I couldn't do anything. This left it all up to my brother. He's been the black sheep of the family—drinks heavily, divorced, etc. and he had not been on very good terms with Dad. I was afraid he couldn't handle things properly. This really bothered me—(Begins to cry openly. Slight pause.)	
(I got up and partially closed the curtains around Mr. Wilson's bed.)	This is shameful—to cry. A grown man shouldn't do this—should be able to control it.	
It is all right to cry, Mr. Wilson.	(Continues to cry. Does not seem able to speak. Continues for approximately 1-2 minutes.)	
(I sat quietly in the chair)	(Wiping eyes.) I'm sorry, but these things have just been building up.	
Sometimes it's good to express them.	Yes, I was so worried that my brother would not be able to take care of things, but my sister said he did very well. Maybe, at last he reconciled himself with Dad. They were never very close. I know this bothered Dad. I was always closest to my father. Things happened so suddenly, it's going to take some getting used to. I will miss him a great deal. But now, maybe my brother and I can be closer. (Pause. Mr. Wilson has stopped crying.) It feels good to talk about this. I think I was just bottling everything up inside. Would you like some candy?	
No, thank you. I am glad to be able to talk with you. I have to leave now, but I will be back to see you before I leave at 12.	Fine. Thank you Miss Baker. (Smiles.)	

YOUR ANSWER

3. a.

    b.

    c.

4. a.

   b.

   c.

CORRECT ANSWER

3. a. Miss Baker used clues she had about what he might be feeling from her general knowledge about what a person would be likely to feel if his parent had died and he was unable to be there or to attend the funeral.
   b. She looked closely for clues from his face or voice.
   c. She used statements of fact to encourage him to go on rather than assuming what he might be feeling.
4. a. Miss Baker provided privacy by closing the curtains.
   b. She explicitly accepts the expression of feeling.
   c. She phrased her comments in such a way that he was encouraged to go on when it appeared that he was ready to express feelings.

219

In the following interaction between Mrs. Drucker and Miss Sanders, look specifically at Miss Sanders' responses numbered 1 through 4 and Mrs. Drucker's comment following each of those responses, then state:
   a. Whether the nurses response is useful or not.
   b. If not useful, state a preferable response.

Interaction Between Mrs. Drucker and Miss Sanders.
Miss S: "Mrs. Drucker?"
Mrs. D: "Yes."
Miss S: "Good morning. I'm Miss Sanders, a sophomore student nurse and I'm going to help you this morning."
Mrs. D: "That will be fine." (Continues to eat breakfast.)
Miss S: "How is your breakfast?"
Mrs. D: "Oh, it's fine. I guess I'll drink the milk instead of the coffee. Milk is more nutritional, isn't it?"
Miss S: "More nutritional?"
Mrs. D: "I mean more than coffee."
Miss S: "Yes. It has more food value."
Mrs. D: "I always get so many liquids. I feel like I have to choose between them since I can't possibly drink them all. Do they want you to drink a lot of liquids after an operation?"
Miss S: "You should, because you are in bed and not moving much, and fluids help to keep your kidneys flushed out." (1)
Mrs. D: "Oh, I see. I'll try to drink all I can, then."
Miss S: (Pause) "Did you sleep well last night?"
Mrs. D: "No, I didn't. I had an awful night. I woke up in the morning and I couldn't move so I called the nurse and she couldn't move me either, so she stayed with me until I got some pills and finally fell asleep. This morning I woke up and could move again."
Miss S: "How do you feel now?"
Mrs. D: "I feel so stiff and weak all over."
Miss S: "All over?"
Mrs. D: "Yes, just everywhere."

Miss S: "Um-hmm. (Pause) Do you want me to leave so you can finish eating or shall I stay?" (2)

Mrs. D: (Still eating) "Oh, stay and just talk to me."

Miss S: "All right." (Pulls up chair and sits down.) (3)

Mrs. D: (Pause) "Oh, I feel so . . . so . . . ."

Miss S: "So what?"

Mrs. D: "So listless." (Becoming tearful) "It all started in the night."

Miss S: "What happened?"

Mrs. D: "I had these awful nightmares."

Miss S: "You had nightmares?"

Mrs. D: "Yes, they were just terrible. You see I've always had this fear of being paralyzed and now my arm is so stiff. The doctor said my nerve was pinched during the operation, but with exercise I should be able to use it completely again."

Miss S: "How far can you move it?"

Mrs. D: "I'm supposed to touch my left ear, like this."

Miss S: "That was very good. You seem to be able to move it quite well."

Mrs. D: "The doctors say I'm doing very well, but I just don't feel much better."

Miss S: "It hasn't been long since your operation and you are moving your arm very well." (4)

Mrs. D: "Yes. (Pause) Do you think I could get up after I eat?"

YOUR ANSWER

  1.

  2.

  3.

  4.

CORRECT ANSWER

  1. Useful
  2. a. Not useful
     b. "Describe how you feel," or "Tell me more about how you feel."
  3. Useful
  4. a. Not useful
     b. "How do you think you should be doing?"

BEHAVIORAL OBJECTIVE:

When the patient begins the process of problem solving, the student helps the patient to define the situation and provides information that will help the patient to cope realistically with the problem. (Frames 220–241)

220

In the interactions with Mr. Wilson and Mrs. Drucker the nurse has been primarily concerned with encouraging the patient to express his feelings since this tends to reduce tension and anxiety. At the same time, the patient may begin to work through a problem.

Read the three different patient responses below. In each response, the patient has stated initially, "I wonder if I'll ever go back to work." The nurse replies, "What has the doctor said about your returning to work?"

Patient Response

1. "The doctor thinks that my leg won't be completely cured. I've been a window washer all my life, and he says it would be dangerous for me to go back to working in high places. I guess maybe he's right."

2. "He says I'm really getting along fine. Nephritis isn't a fatal disease, and I will undoubtedly be able to go back to work, but somehow I can't stop worrying about it."

3. "Well, he told me that within six months I probably won't be around any more. I guess I've got to accept that I won't be going back to work."

(Go on to the next frame.)

221

In the example below, we have extended one of the conversations from the previous frame.

1. What has the nurse done in this conversation?
2. What effect has her action had?

Patient: "I wonder if I'll ever go back to work?"

Nurse: "What has the doctor said about you returning to work?"

Patient: "The doctor thinks that my leg won't be completely cured. I've been a window washer all my life, and he says it would be dangerous for me to go back to working in high places. I guess maybe he's right."

Nurse: "You agree that going on as a window washer might be too risky?"

Patient: "Uh, huh. It's hard to change jobs so late in life, but I've got to think of something else to do."

Nurse: "You're thinking about other possibilities?"

Patient: "I have a brother who said he might fix me up with work, or I can get a couple of interviews after I'm home.

(Conversation continues)

YOUR ANSWER

CORRECT ANSWER

1. The nurse has encouraged the patient to express his thoughts and feelings about returning to work.

2. It has given the patient the opportunity to begin to work through his problem.

222

Frequently, a patient may seek to solve problems with the assistance of the nurse. For example, he may have to decide whether or not to have surgery, think of ways to reduce the demands of his work, or plan changes in his diet that are required by doctor's orders. In these situations the decisions are ultimately the patient's decisions. The nurse can help the patient to express his feelings, to clarify his feelings, and to consider possible alternative actions. She may also at times provide information.

(Go on to the next frame.)

223

You are Lauren Nichols, a 24 year old woman who is an artist. You have worked for two years on the staff of a national magazine as an illustrator. This July you are scheduled to have your first art show at a local gallery. You have been working diligently getting ready for this, but you still have several paintings to complete to meet your contractual agreement for the show.

Three days ago, on February 13th, you fell on the ice and suffered a compound fracture of your right arm. It is now in a cast which will be on your arm for eight weeks. The doctor has told you that it will be at least two months after the cast is removed before you regain normal functioning of your arm.

Try to imagine the specific feelings you would have and list them below.

YOUR ANSWER

CORRECT ANSWER

Your answer may have included:
1. Frustration
2. Helplessness
3. Anger
4. Depression

224

Read Interaction I between Lauren and Miss Dykstra. Imagine yourself as Lauren.

Interaction I Between Lauren Nichols and Miss Dykstra

It is now midafternoon and you, as Lauren, are looking absently out the window, thinking about your problems and reflecting upon the sudden change that has come into your life. Miss Dykstra, a nurse, enters the room and the following conversation occurs.

Miss D: "Hello, Lauren. I'd like to check the circulation in your fingers."
Lauren: (Sighs) "Oh . . . Well, I don't see that there's much point in it, but all right, go ahead."
Miss D: "Okay, just put your arm over here and I'll check it. (Pause) (Cheerfully) It seems to be coming along nicely."
Lauren: "I guess *that* all depends on your point of view."
Miss D: Your arm will be healed soon and everything will be all right again.
Lauren: "Well, maybe that would be all right for most people, but it isn't for me!"
Miss D: "How is it different for you?"
Lauren: "Four months before I can use my arm again! I've got things to do before then!"
Miss D: "Sometimes we have to delay our plans. Four months isn't really very long."
Lauren: "But I have a commitment to keep and now I won't be able to keep it. I'm supposed to have these paintings ready. The gallery owner . . . ."
Miss D: (Interrupting) "Well, I think you'll find that when you're dealing with people, most of them will make allowances. I don't think you should worry about this now. Just look at the brighter side: your arm is going to heal and you will be able to paint. It will just be on into the future.

Lauren: (Voice rising) "You just don't understand! This is terribly important to me!"

Miss D: "I'm sure you'll work out this problem, Lauren. The important thing now is that the circulation in your hand is not impaired and healing has already begun."

What kinds of feelings do you, as Lauren, have now?

YOUR ANSWER

CORRECT ANSWER

Your answers may vary somewhat, but one person's answers were as follows.

1. I'm angry because it's obvious that Miss Dykstra doesn't have any understanding about me as an individual, the kind of person I am, and what kind of life plans and commitments I have.

2. I feel more depressed and more alone, as though I'm in the hospital without any help available at all. So I feel even more helpless.

3. I feel frustrated, not only by the situation but by the fact that there's no understanding.

All of the feelings that I felt before are intensified.

225

A. What do you think was Lauren's primary concern during the preceding conversation?

YOUR ANSWER

CORRECT ANSWER

Her preoccupation with the status of her career *now* and the effects of her injury on the development of her career.

B. What do you think were Miss Dykstra's goals during the preceding conversation?

YOUR ANSWER

CORRECT ANSWER

1. To make a physical assessment; that is, to check the circulation in Lauren's fingers.
2. To cheer Lauren and try to define her injury as a minor interruption in her life.

C. What do you think Miss Dykstra's goals should have been?

YOUR ANSWER

CORRECT ANSWER

The first goal would have remained the same.

The second would be to encourage Lauren to express her feelings and begin to work through her problem, if she wished.

226

Now read Interaction II between Lauren and Miss McDonald. Again imagine yourself as Lauren.

Interaction II Between Lauren Nichols and Miss McDonald

Miss M: "Hello, Lauren. I'd like to check the circulation in your fingers."

Lauren: (Sighs) "Oh . . . okay."

Miss M: "Okay, just put your arm over here and I'll check it. (Pause) (Cheerfully) The circulation looks fine. Things seem to be coming along well."

Lauren: "Hmmm. (Discouraged) That all depends on your point of view."

Miss M: "Well, what is your point of view?"

Lauren: "Well, I suppose that the circulation may be all right. It may be that everything's going normally, but I have an art show scheduled for July. I'll never have those paintings ready in four months!"

Miss M: "This accident has really put a crimp in your plans, hasn't it?"

Lauren: "Yeah, I don't really see any way out of it . . . ."

Miss M: "Your show is scheduled for July and this accident will keep you from completing the paintings in time."

Lauren: "Yes. That much is certain. I *hate* this feeling of not being able to *do* anything! . . . And, you know what else? I haven't gotten up my courage to call the gallery to tell them I broke my arm!"

Miss M: "You're worried about their reaction."

Lauren: "Yes. They'll have to cancel my show and I don't know if they'll *ever* be able to show my work!"

Miss M: "Is their whole schedule worked out that many months in advance?"

Lauren: "I don't know. It was hard to schedule my show in the first place."

Miss M: "What do you think the gallery will say when you tell them what happened to you?"

Lauren: "Well, they have their own commitment to make too, and they'd have to arrange another show. I suppose they might try to get another artist to show at that time. Then there are two possibilities: they'd forget all about my show or, under the circumstances, they might set another date later on."

Miss M: So you want to find out what their decision is."

Lauren: "Yes! That is something that I can do, and I may as well do it right now. Would you pleas set the telephone over here closer to me?"

What kinds of feelings do you, as Lauren, have now?

YOUR ANSWER

CORRECT ANSWER

1. I was able to express my feelings of anger and frustration at the accident.
2. I feel less hopeless because I see some action I can take.
3. Miss McDonald has seen me as a particular person with a definite kind of life plan which has been disrupted.

227

A. What do you think was Lauren's primary concern during the preceding conversation?

YOUR ANSWER

CORRECT ANSWER

1. Her preoccupation with the status of her career *now* and the effects of her injury on the de development of her career.
2. Trying to find out the most effective way to deal with the current problem.

B. What do you think was Miss McDonald's goal during the preceding conversation?

YOUR ANSWER

CORRECT ANSWER

1. To make a physical assessment; that is, to check the circulation in Lauren's fingers.
2. To encourage Lauren to express her feelings and begin to work through her problem, if she wished.

228

The patient, Mrs. Carson, is sitting slumped in the chair beside her bed. She is staring at the floor with wide, unblinking eyes. The nurse enters briskly. In the following interaction between Mrs. Carson and Miss Bartel, notice each of Miss Bartel's comments (numbered 1 through 3) and:

   a.   Determine whether the nurse's response is useful or not.
   b.   If not useful, state a preferable response.

Interaction I Between Mrs. Carson and Miss Bartel

Nurse: "Oh, come now, Mrs. Carson! Nothing can be *that* bad! You look as if you've just lost your last friend." (1)

Mrs. Carson: "The doctor told me that it will be impossible for me to get well if I don't have the operation! (said breathlessly) I'm so mixed up! I wish I knew what to do!"

Nurse: "There's only one thing to do, and that is to have the surgery. You haven't a thing to worry about! You have the best surgeon in town. He's done hundreds of operations just like yours!" (2)

Mrs. Carson: "You don't understand! I *have* confidence in my doctor's skill, it's . . . well . . . it's . . . "

Nurse: (Interrupting) "Most people are frightened of having an operation. Remember when you had your baby several years ago while I was working on OB? You had the longest and hardest labor of anyone on the ward, and I never heard a whimper out of you. I was so proud of you! You were the best patient in the whole hospital. After what you went through, this operation would be a picnic! This time you'll be completely unconscious from the anesthetic. You won't feel a thing!" (3)

YOUR ANSWER

   1.

   2.

   3.

CORRECT ANSWER

   1. a.   Not useful
      b.   "You look as though something is bothering you."
   2. a.   Not useful
      b.   "Is there some problem with you having the surgery?"
   3. a.   Not useful
      b.   (If Miss Bartel doesn't interrupt, Mrs. Carson might say it herself.)
           "What is the important thing then, Mrs. Carson?"

229

Miss Bartel was ineffective in her interaction with Mrs. Carson. What three things caused her ineffectiveness?

YOUR ANSWER

1.

2.

3.

CORRECT ANSWER

1. Miss Bartel implies that it is inappropriate for Mrs. Carson to have the feelings she does.
2. She doesn't try to find out what is bothering Mrs. Carson, she assumes she knows.
3. On the basis of her assumptions, she gives advice.

230

Later in the day another nurse, Miss Franco, enters Mrs. Carson's room. Mrs. Carson is lying in bed, staring into space. Her cheeks are tear-stained. After a preliminary greeting, the nurse asks Mrs. Carson to turn over so she can rub her back. As Mrs. Carson complies, a conversation takes place. When you have read Interaction II between Mrs. Carson and Miss Franco, answer the questions lettered A through D.

Interaction II Between Mrs. Carson and Miss Franco

Nurse: "It seems hard for you to relax tonight. You must've had a difficult day."

Mrs. Carson: (Quietly) "Yes."

Nurse: "Would you like to tell me about it?"

Mrs. Carson: (Hesitantly) "It would seem silly to you. It's so hard to explain. If I thought I could make it home, I would leave! No one understands!"

Nurse: (Kindly) "I would like to try to understand if it will help you."

Mrs. Carson: "They say I have to have another operation and I'm *so* scared and mixed up! They think it's the operation that scares me but . . . oh, well, I don't know if you could understand. I'm such a mess!"

Nurse: "It's hard to talk about it?"

Mrs. Carson: "Yes, if I weren't around, maybe he could get someone who would really help John. I just don't have the patience any more. Maybe I never did!"

Nurse: "Could you tell me who John is, and *who* could get someone else?"

Mrs. Carson: "John is my oldest child. He has cerebral palsy. He's a sweet little boy, but he needs so much care and you have to be so patient with him, and I'm just not! Since I've been sick, we haven't been able to send him to a special school. My medical bills stand in the way of his chances to get help and when he's home all the time, I guess I get impatient with his troubles and I'm always scolding when I know he can't help it. My husband has the burden of both of us. He is so kind to the boy and so patient with me. They'd both be better off without me! I shouldn't have the operation!"

Nurse: "Are you saying that you may not live if you don't have the operation and that this would be better for John and for your husband?"

Mrs. Carson: "The doctor said that I can't expect to live long if I don't have surgery. I guess I am really silly! That would be kind of like suicide, wouldn't it? Now you know how mixed up I am! (sniff) I guess I'm a little crazy, worrying about John and the money and everything."

Nurse:	"It's such a tough problem that you would just like to escape from it."
Mrs. Carson:	"Yes, but I don't really want to die! I can't really say that my husband would be better off if I were to die! He'd be all alone with our little boy. What a coward I am! What would he do all alone? And Johnny! He needs me even if I'm not much of a mother right at the moment. If I just knew what to do! If I could be just patient like the other mothers."
Nurse:	"All mothers get angry and impatient with their children sometimes."
Mrs. Carson:	"I do get angry at the other children. But I don't feel so bad when I jump on them."
Nurse:	"It's more difficult with John, because he has special problems."
Mrs. Carson:	"Yes, I feel so helpless with John. I guess if I knew how to work with him better, I wouldn't be so impatient."
Nurse:	"We have a specially trained person on our staff who works with children with cerebral palsy. She might be helpful to you and to John. If you feel you'd like to talk with her, it could be arranged."
Mrs. Carson:	"Yes, I would! I used to talk with John's teacher and that helped a lot. But since he hasn't been in school I haven't seen her. We must get him back in school soon. We'll have to borrow money for the operation and that's why his schooling has to wait. I wish that there was some way to pay for both at the same time."
Nurse:	"Perhaps one of our social workers could talk with you about your financial problems, and you could make some arrangements so they wouldn't be such a burden to you."
Mrs. Carson:	"I'd like my husband to see the social worker with me. Could we do it before the operation?"
Nurse:	"I'm sure that could be arranged. (Smiles) You look a little more comfortable now. I'll be back in a few moments with some medication for you."

A. Miss Franco tries to understand Mrs. Carson's situation as she sees it. Cite examples of this.

YOUR ANSWER

CORRECT ANSWER

1. Because Mrs. Carson seems pre-occupied and has tear-stained cheeks, Miss Franco tries to ascertain the reason for this with her initial statement.
2. Miss Franco says, "Would you like to tell me about it?"
3. She asks, "Who is John?" and "Who could get someone else?"

B. Miss Franco provides information to help Mrs. Carson begin to solve her problems. Cite examples of this.

YOUR ANSWER

CORRECT ANSWER

1. She tells Mrs. Carson that the social worker will be able to talk with her and her husband about their financial problems.

2. She promises to make arrangements for Mrs. Carson to talk with a trained person about her problems with her son, Johnny.

C. Miss Franco accepts Mrs. Carson's feelings. Cite examples of this.

YOUR ANSWER

CORRECT ANSWER

1. "You must've had a difficult day."
2. "I would like to try to understand."
3. "It's hard to talk about it?"

D. Miss Franco checks with Mrs. Carson, or validates with her that she has received her message correctly. Cite example of this.

YOUR ANSWER

CORRECT ANSWER

1. "Are you saying that you may not live if you don't have the operation and that this would be better for John and your husband?"
2. "It's such a tough problem that you would just like to escape from it."
3. "It's more difficult with John because he has special problems."

231

If you look at the two interactions with Mrs. Carson, it is obvious that in the first one she felt frustrated because she was misinterpreted. In the second, she felt relieved that she was able to express her feelings and have them understood and accepted. She also felt relieved because she found some solutions to her problems.

(Go on to the next frame.)

232

Mrs. Georgine Black is 37 years old. Her husband, Larry, is a tenant farmer in Ohio. They have seven children, ranging in age from three to fifteen. Three years ago they moved from Southern Kentucky to Southern Ohio. As a child, Mrs. Black had rheumatic fever, which left her with rheumatic heart disease. In recent years her condition has been growing worse and Mrs. Black developed congestive heart failure. She came to the hospital for evaluation and possible surgery. Three weeks ago she had her aortic valve replaced. This present hospitalization was paid for by the Heart Fund.

Mrs. Black is getting ready to go home in about four or five days. It will be several months before she is able to resume normal activity. Mrs. Mercer has been one of the nurses caring for Mrs. Black since her admission. Mrs. Mercer will be helping to prepare Mrs. Black for her return home in order that her convalescence will go as smoothly as possible.

On the basis of the information given above, what problems might you anticipate when Mrs. Black returns home?

YOUR ANSWER

CORRECT ANSWER

She has a great deal of responsibility (having seven children) and few financial resources. Therefore, it will be difficult for her to rest as much as she should.

233

On the basis of the problems you anticipate, what would Mrs. Mercer want to find out in order to help Mrs. Black?

YOUR ANSWER

CORRECT ANSWER

1. Who might she possibly have to help her care for her children?
2. a. What is her attitude toward her illness and her long convalescent period?
   b. What is her attitude toward having people help her?
3. What does she know about the activity she will be allowed during her convalescence?

234

As you read the following interaction between Mrs. Black and Mrs. Mercer, keep in mind the three questions that you should have identified at the end of the preceding frame. You will be asked to provide answers to those questions, derived from this interaction.

Interaction I Between Mrs. Black and Mrs. Mercer

Mrs. Black: "Oh, hi there, Mrs. Mercer."

Mrs. Mercer: "Good morning, Mrs. Black. How are you this morning?"

Mrs. Black: (With enthusiasm) "Oh, I feel *real* good this morning. You know, I got up just a little while ago and I walked to the bathroom, and I felt pretty good. I got there and my legs were just a little bit wobbly."

Mrs. Mercer: "I suppose if you build up to it kind of gradually and if you go once this morning and once this afternoon, you will probably be getting some of your strength back.

Mrs. Black: "Yeh, well . . . the Doctor, he won't let me get up but once or twice a day, but at least I get to go to the bathroom now instead of having to use the 'pan.' "

Mrs. Mercer: "Uh-huh, are you getting ready to go home pretty soon?"

Mrs. Black: "Yes, you know I think I will be going home in about 4 days, on Saturday that is. Doctor said if everything goes along like it has been, that I will be able to go home then."

Mrs. Mercer: "Has he had any talks with you about what you will be able to do when you go home? As far as activities are concerned."

Mrs. Black: "Uh . . . not real specifically, he told me that I had to stay in bed for at least a couple of weeks, then gradually work back into my regular housework, and that kind of stuff. Uh, I guess that uh, he says that if I didn't do this and when I went back, I started right back on working hard again, I could undo-all the surgery they did, and he spoke kinda serious about it. And you know, he said that my heart was still weak where they put this valve in and if I worked too hard my heart would pump too hard, and it would just blow out this valve. And it would blow up, and I could die. And he also said if I worked too hard and I'm kind of thin, and uh . . . I'm weak still . . . I might get an infection and he said the first place that infection would go is right around that valve. And if it goes to that valve it would weaken it and it might blow up again, and I could die, immediately."

Mrs. Mercer: "Well, that's kind of frightening to think about, isn't it?"

Mrs. Black: (Quickly) "Yes it is, and you know . . . I thought everything was over, you know!"

Mrs. Mercer: "Uh-huh!"

Mrs. Black: "And, uh, and I thought I was through worrying about that, but he said it could still happen, and this is why I have to mind myself at home and pace myself."

Mrs. Mercer: "Uh-huh, uh-huh. Are you still concerned that you might get an infection? Or that, as you said, you heart might blow the valve out?"

Mrs. Black: "Well . . . (pause) . . . I thought about it, because I was thinkin about, you know, what I'm a-goin' to have to be doin' at home. You see, I've got 7 children and uh, most of 'um are in school, but I've got 3 year old Billy and he is still at home, and there is an awful lot of stuff to be done at home, and uh . . . I was just thinkin about how I was going to get all of the stuff done . . . and I kinda have to get around a little bit more and do some more housework . . . that kind of stuff. (Pause) I don't think . . . . I had my surgery for my children."

Mrs. Mercer: "Uh-huh"

Mrs. Black: "And the Doctors told me I wouldn't live without the surgery, they said that uh . . . if I did have the surgery I might die, there was a 50/50 chance that I could live and I made the decision to go through with it for my children . . . because I thought, they need a mother, and they haven't had one for awhile, 'cause I've been really sick. And I haven't been doin' too much at home but stayin' in bed and that stuff, and that's why I had the surgery."

Mrs. Mercer: "So you feel that you kind of have resolved it in your own mind, that you had the surgery so you wouldn't die, and now even though there is a chance that if you did get an infection, then you have done what you thought was best . . . to have the surgery."

Mrs. Black: "That's right, the Good Lord willin', I'm goin' to be O.K., and uh, I made it over the one hump of surgery, and I'm not too afraid of actually dying . . . I don't think . . . I worried about that enough before the surgery, but I really do think that I uh, I will be O.K. once I get home."

Mrs. Mercer: "You mentioned your 3 year old little boy—is someone taking care of him now?"

Mrs. Black: "Yes. Right now my sister is, she lives . . . oh, just a little ways down the road and she has 4 youngins of her own, but she takes care of my Billy. My husband, he drops him off at her house on the way to work in the morning, and then picks him up in the evening when he comes back. And she has done a *real* nice job of takin' care of him."

Mrs. Mercer: "Well, that's nice that she has been so close."

Mrs. Black: (Quickly) "Yes!"

Mrs. Mercer: "And she has been able to do it!"

Mrs. Black: "Well, she is a real sweet girl, she has tried to help me out all she could."

Mrs. Mercer: "Are your other children all in school? How old is the oldest?"

Mrs. Black: "Uh, she is 15, that's my first."

Mrs. Mercer: "She's old enough to have helped you out through all of this, isn't she?"

Mrs. Black: "Oh yes! I must say that she was, even before I came into the hospital. You know, I couldn't do anything . . . I was in bed most of the day, and my Susie, she just did . . . she just did marvelous. You know she cooked the meals, all the meals, and made sure everyone got fed right. And she cleaned the house, or supervised it at least, she had the other children helping her, but she just done a wonderful job, and I guess she has been doin' the same thing since I was in the hospital.

Mrs. Mercer: "Uh-huh!"

Mrs. Black: "I don't know . . . I haven't seen her."

Mrs. Mercer: "Uh-huh."

Mrs. Black: "I kinda miss 'em because I haven't seen any of them since I have been here."

Mrs. Mercer: "Oh! You haven't?"

Mrs. Black: (Somewhat sadly) "No."

Mrs. Mercer: "Well, how far away do you live?"

Mrs. Black: "Oh, I guess it is about, uh, oh probably 200 miles from here, 180 miles, it's in the southern part of Ohio."

Mrs. Mercer: "Oh yes, that would be a long way for them to come."

Mrs. Black: "Yes, my husband, he comes every week-end, every Saturday, to see me, but uh, he can't bring the children cause he can't bring them up here, with the little boy, and I can't go down-stairs to see them, so there is no use in bringin' them."

Mrs. Mercer: "Well . . . now getting back to when you go home, has the Doctor talked to you, more specifically about what activities he would like you to do when you are home? At first?

Mrs. Black: "Well . . . (pause) . . . what he told me, was that I couldn't do anything, that I would have to take to the bed for the first two weeks, and I couldn't do anything and then after that, he said that I could work an hour a day, but I had to do 'light work.' Uh, I'm not sure what that is."

Mrs. Mercer: "Did he say what light work was?"

Mrs. Black: "No . . . (pause) . . . no, I . . . I imagine it means like setting the table, or peeling the potatoes for supper, or something like that. Uh, I suppose that is what he means.

Mrs. Mercer: "Something that you could probably do sitting down and not moving around?"

Mrs. Black: "Yes, yes, that is what I suppose light work is, and then after that, each week, I could add an hour on a day. And the whole deal, uh, might take about 4 or 6 months. I guess! Before I could get back to what I was doin' before."

Mrs. Mercer: "Gee, that is quite a while, isn't it? For you to convalesce?"

Mrs. Black: "Yes, it is quite a while, but uh, I suppose I had better do what the Doctor says."

Now write your answers to the questions that were identified at the end of the preceding frame:

YOUR ANSWER

1. (Resources for family care)

2. (Mrs. Black's attitude toward her illness)

3. (Her knowledge of allowed activities)

CORRECT ANSWER

1. Her sister, and Susie, her oldest child.
2. a. Mrs. Black seems to realize that since she's gone through the surgery she should follow the doctor's orders.
   b. She seems grateful for the help of Susie and her sister.
3. She knows that she has to stay in bed for two weeks, then increase her activity one hour per day. She can do light work, but is unsure of what that really means.
She knows that if she overworks she could "blow out her valve" and die.
She knows that if she overworks and gets weak she might get sick and have an infection around her valve.

235

Read Interaction II between Mrs. Black and Mrs. Mercer, which is a continuation of the preceding conversation and in which you will find out additional and conflicting information about Mrs. Black's problems. You will again be asked to provide answers to the questions which end the two preceding frames.

Interaction II Between Mrs. Black and Mrs. Mercer

Mrs. Mercer: "Do you feel that you will be able to do it when you get home?"

Mrs. Black: "Well, well, (pause) I suppose, if I have to . . . that I can do it. (Pause) See what the problem is, that I have this 3 year old son, and uh, 3 year olds run around a lot. And they do a lot of stuff and I . . . I just don't see how I can stay in bed, and keep an eye on Billy.

Mrs. Mercer: "Uh-huh"

Mrs. Black: "We only got 3 rooms, but still I can be in the bedroom and he can be somewhere else and . . ."

Mrs. Mercer: "Is there anyone that can help you look after Billy? When you get home."

Mrs. Black: "Well . . . my sister I suppose (with question in her voice) but she has been lookin' after him for such a long time, because she helped me when I was so sick before, and I couldn't go to the hospital, and she does have 4 youngins of her own, and 2 at home, with 2 in school. And I think she has her hands full, and I kinda hate to ask her to do it for me."

Mrs. Mercer: "Do you think it might be an imposition on her, if you asked her?"

Mrs. Black: "Yes, I do!"

Mrs. Mercer: "Well, you said you lived out in the country. How close is this to a town?"

Mrs. Black: "Oh, about 4 or 5 miles from a little town . . . .

Mrs. Mercer: "But there is a 'Visiting Nurses Association,' where there might be people who could come out and help you for ½ day twice a week, or something like that."

Mrs. Black: "Oh, I didn't know that!"

Mrs. Mercer: "You might be able to look into that here, before you leave for home and see what is available so you could get some help."

Mrs. Black: "Well, that . . . well that is something. I didn't know about that. Would . . . would it cost any money?"

Mrs. Mercer: "I'm not really sure, I would have to talk with someone from the Social Services here, or from the Visiting Nurses Association, to see, but I will check on it, if you like. Then I'll come back and tell you what I found out."

Mrs. Black: "Oh! (Enthusiastically) That sounds good."

Mrs. Mercer: (Smiles)

Mrs. Black: "That sounds like a good idea, you know, I also . . . thinkin' about the whole thing, I was kind of worried about my children having to work so hard for me, because. . . well . . . you know that Susie of mine, she's in High School and she is doin' *real good* in High School and she is going to finish, I think. And that's *real* important. I . . . I wasn't much interested, and I didn't finish the 8th grade, but my Susie she likes school, and she seems to be doin' real good. And she's got a lot of friends, but she *NEVER* sees them, except at school, and she is so busy with takin' care of things at home, that she, uh, can't go out at night and see 'em, and she can't go out on the week-ends, she has got to clean and cook, and . . . help the children, and look out after them. But my husband, he works, he works on Sundays usually, he gets Saturdays off to come up here but he's not around too much to help and uh . . . ."

Mrs. Mercer: (Interrupting) "So you think this might be a problem when you get home? That Susie will still be doing a lot of the work?"

Mrs. Black: "Yes, and then, she hasn't complained about it or anything. Well, uh, when I was her age, I wanted to be with my friends, and do things with them. And I didn't spend much time at home, and Susie hasn't been able to do any of that. Uh, she has been so busy at home, that uh, well . . . I feel badly for her."

Mrs. Mercer: "Uh-huh . . . ."

Mrs. Black: "Well, I think an awful lot of her, and she has been an awful good girl to me, and helped me out so much, and she is just wonderful, but I think she ought to have some kinda life of her own and uh . . . her schoolin' too. I don't know how much longer she can sit up nights with the kids a-screamin' and she use to want to go to the library at night and stuff, and see her friends there and do her homework. But, she can't do that now . . . and uh . . . well I don't think that's good for her at all."

Mrs. Mercer: "Well, have you thought about this—what you might do when you get home?"

Mrs. Black: "Well . . . to tell you the truth, I uh . . . wasn't plannin' uh . . . on exactly doin' what the Doctor said. I thought that I would try and take it easy, but I'd have little Billy with me, and I'd have to keep an eye on him . . . ."

Mrs. Mercer: "Uh-hum."

Mrs. Black: " . . . and keep him out of trouble and all that stuff and I thought that . . . well, that I'd, you know . . . that I'd start plannin' the meals and I'd . . . well I wouldn't move furniture or that kinda stuff, now I know I couldn't do that . . . but I was thinkin' that I could go at it slow, but . . . that I'd kinda go back and be a mother and housewife again.

Now write your answers to the questions that were identified at the ends of the preceding two frames:

YOUR ANSWER

1. (Resources for family care)

2. (Mrs. Black's attitude toward her illness)

3. (Her knowledge of allowed activities)

CORRECT ANSWER

1. Mrs. Black is reluctant to burden her sister and daughter with continued responsibility for her family, even though they themselves are not reluctant, as far as we know. The Visiting Nurse is a possible resource.

2. Because she doesn't want to burden others, she is going back to her original schedule, avoiding only the most strenuous work.

3. This remains the same.

236

Read Interaction III between Mrs. Black and Mrs. Mercer, which is a continuation of the preceding conversation.

Interaction III Between Mrs. Black and Mrs. Mercer

Mrs. Mercer: "Well this is a pretty serious decision in terms of some of the consequences it might have for you, isn't it?"

Mrs. Black: "Well, I haven't thought too much about it, to tell you the truth ... I ... just figured the Good Lord took care of me this far and He'd take care of me even farther ...."

Mrs. Mercer: "Uh-hum."

Mrs. Black: " ... when I get home."

Mrs. Mercer: "Does your family know anything about what you've decided? Do they know that you are not going to abide by some of the strict rest regulations and working regulations?"

Mrs. Black: "No. No, I ... last time I saw my husband I didn't know, and the Doctor just told me a couple of days ago."

Mrs. Mercer: "Uh-huh."

Mrs. Black: "So, uh, no I didn't tell them."

Mrs. Mercer: "Oh, well, I wonder how they might feel about this?"

Mrs. Black: (Silence)

Mrs. Mercer: "You know, you have said several times how good they have been and they have pitched in to help and to do all of the work? And they want you back there as well as you can be, and I wonder how they would feel if they thought you might be undoing some of the things that you had done here, with the surgery."

Mrs. Black: "Well, I don't know I ... well I was kinda afraid to tell 'em ... matter of fact ... I wasn't goin' to say anything about what the Doctor said.

Mrs. Mercer: "Oh!"

Mrs. Black: "I was goin' to kinda modify what the Doctor said, I guess."

Mrs. Mercer: "Oh."

Mrs. Black: "Actually, if I think about it, though, I guess that, as I said before, I had that surgery for my children because they need a mother ... and uh ... I wouldn't be any good to them dead. And uh ... if I go home and do too much, I guess, I could die anyway, and I wouldn't be any good to them, and why go through all of this stuff with the surgery, if ... I'm just going to undo it all."

Remember that the first comment Mrs. Mercer made in Interaction II was, "Do you feel that you will be able to do it when you get home?"

Mrs. Mercer's first comment in Interaction III is, "This is a pretty serious decision in terms of some of the consequences it might have for you, isn't it?"

What is the goal of both of these comments?

YOUR ANSWER

CORRECT ANSWER

To encourage Mrs. Black to examine the realities of her own situation.

237

Mrs. Black has stated that she is not going to follow the doctor's orders when she gets home. Mrs. Mercer knows, and Mrs. Black really knows, too, that this would endanger her life. When Mrs. Mercer says, "This is a pretty serious decision for you in terms of some of the consequences it might have for you, isn't it?" Mrs. Mercer hopes that these consequences will convince Mrs. Black to follow the doctor's regimen.

1. What is the major reason for Mrs. Black's reluctance to follow the doctor's regimen?

YOUR ANSWER

CORRECT ANSWER

She doesn't want to burden her eldest daughter and her sister with any more responsibility.

2. What does Mrs. Mercer know specifically about Mrs. Black's life goals that will help her in the conversation?

YOUR ANSWER

CORRECT ANSWER

She knows that Mrs. Black is devoted to her children and had the surgery so that she would have a better chance of remaining alive to take care of them.

238

Read Interaction IV, a continuation of the preceding conversation and see how Mrs. Mercer uses these ideas in talking with Mrs. Black.

Interaction IV Between Mrs. Black and Mrs. Mercer

Mrs. Mercer: "Well, I think that's right. You did say that they are all helping you, and that the older ones, as well as Susan, were doing some of the chores around the house, didn't you?"

Mrs. Black: "Oh, yes."

Mrs. Mercer: "Have you thought at all about maybe dividing up some of the chores, so that it would be more of a scheduled thing, or they would know more of what they were going to do? Instead of saying, well, you know, I'll just pitch in—that can be pretty indefinite. And with you home they might not pitch in as much, but if you had a schedule, perhaps, or had something worked out where each one knew what they were doing . . . you know, it might be different."

Mrs. Black: "I see what you mean, (with enthusiasm) like write down what each child should do . . . ."

Mrs. Mercer: "Yes."

Mrs. Black: "In the way of chores, and then . . . maybe put it up on the wall, and they could all read it and maybe follow it."

Mrs. Mercer: "Yes, I think it might save you a little bit, you know, rather than thinking 'well, I've got to plan for this one, to do this today,' and if it would be scheduled for a week at a time, it might be easier on you, and easier on them. When they know just what they have to do!"

Mrs. Black: "Yeh, well that sounds like a good idea. Frankly, I . . . hadn't thought about that at all, I . . . thought, well, you know . . . with children, they want to be free, and I know the younger ones try and get out of this, cause Susie told me they did."

Mrs. Mercer: "Uh-huh."

Mrs. Black: "But, maybe, if they had a kinda schedule on the wall, it might be kinda fun for them, too!"

Mrs. Mercer: "Right, at least it might be worth a try, because as you said . . . you did have the surgery so you could be home with them, and be well. You want to stay as well as possible, and not undo all of the good things that were done by the Doctors for the valve in your heart."

Mrs. Black: "That's right . . . that's what I want to do."

Mrs. Mercer: "I'm not exactly sure what the Doctor has in mind as far as light work, I don't really know what he means by 2 hours of moderate work. But I'll talk to him, then I'll come back and perhaps you and I, together, could work out a schedule of what you might be able to do at first, and what each of the children can do. Then you can take it home with you."

Mrs. Black: "Oh, I see."

Mrs. Mercer: "Do you think that might be all right with you?"

Mrs. Black: "That sounds like a good idea . . . I'm . . . I'm . . . sure willing to try. I was kinda afraid to tell you this stuff, 'specially that I wasn't going to follow what the Doctor said. Cause I thought all you would do was kinda tell me that I should do it and . . . ."

Mrs. Mercer: "Uh-huh."

Mrs. Black: (Continues) "But you seem to understand what I'm thinkin' about and the problems with my children and my family."

Mrs. Mercer: "I can appreciate that, because you do want to give them some free time and . . . ."

Mrs. Black: "Yes, I do."

Mrs. Mercer: " . . . and, on the other hand, you don't want to wear yourself out either . . . I think we will be able to work something out, so that, at least, they will have some idea of what has to be done, and you will feel a little more comfortable knowing that these things are being done, and you don't have to see about them being done yourself."

Mrs. Black: "Yes . . . and I suppose I could ask my sister to take care of Billy for a little bit longer, at least until the other children get home from school, then they could look after him."

Mrs. Mercer: "Uh huh."

Mrs. Black: "Cause she is real sweet and, uh . . . I think she would probably help me."

Mrs. Mercer: "Well, we could try that, and I will talk to the people at the Visiting Nurses Association and see what services there are available, near the town—now what is the town that you live near? What is the name of it?

Mrs. Black: "Uh . . . Molene!"

Mrs. Mercer: "O.K. . . . we'll see if we can check on that down there and see what we can come up with, and I'll be back. Probably this afternoon, and we'll talk a little more about the schedule and if we can get anyone to take care of Billy."

Mrs. Black: (Quite enthusiastically) "O.K. Thank you very much!"

Mrs. Mercer: "O.K.—Good-bye."

239

Having now read Interaction IV between Mrs. Black and Mrs. Mercer, answer the following questions:

1. What suggestions did Mrs. Mercer make to Mrs. Black that would lighten the responsibilities of Susie and Mrs. Black's sister?

2. What additional information did Mrs. Mercer need before helping Mrs. Black with her activity schedule.

YOUR ANSWER

1.

2.

CORRECT ANSWER

1. She suggested a work schedule for all of the children in the family.
She would look into the possibility of the Visiting Nurse coming to the house.

2. She needed to find out from the doctor what light work implied.

240

Mrs. Fulton's lunch tray arrived five minutes ago. The nurse, Miss Hughes, passes her bed and notices that Mrs. Fulton has made no effort to begin to eat. In the following interaction between Mrs. Fulton and Miss Hughes, notice each of the nurse's five responses and:

a. Determine whether the nurse's response is useful or not.
b. If not useful, state a preferable response.

Interaction Between Mrs. Nora Fulton and Miss Hughes

Miss H: "Mrs. Fulton, your food will be getting cold. You'd better begin to eat!" (1)

Mrs. F: "I just don't feel like eating today."

Miss H: "What's the matter?" (2)

Mrs. F: "I'm so worried! (Sniffs and begins to cry.) I overheard one of the doctors say this morning that they were going to do some different tests and check for a tumor! You know what *that* means! (Voice rises hysterically) They think I have cancer!"

Miss H: "Oh, no, Mrs. Fulton! There are certain tests that are done on everyone with your problem. Three different ones, I believe." (3)

Mrs. F: "But why didn't the doctors explain that to me? You don't know what it's like to be in here, hardly able to catch my breath and have them whispering among themselves about my symptoms."

Miss H: "That makes you more concerned, then." (4)

Mrs. F: "Yes! I'm too young to be dying of cancer!"

Miss H: "Oh, dear! I think your food has gotten cold. Let me take it back and get you something warmer." (5)

Mrs. F: "Oh . . . (Sniff) Just forget it. I think I'll try to sleep now."

YOUR ANSWER

1.

2.

3.

4.

5.

CORRECT ANSWER

1. a. Not useful
   b. "Is something the matter, Mrs. Fulton?"
2. Useful
3. a. Not useful
   b. "You're worried because the doctors are ordering different tests."
4. Useful
5. a. Not useful.
   b. "You're concerned about dying."

241

In the following interaction between Mr. Robert Holmes and the nurse, Miss Newman, notice each of the nurse's nine responses and:
   a. Determine whether the nurse's response is useful or not.
   b. If not useful, state a preferable response.

Interaction Between Mr. Robert Holmes and Miss Newman

Mr. H: "Oh, nurse! Nurse!"

Miss N: "Yes, Mr. Holmes." (1)

Mr. H: "Would you please move these pillows up behind my back? They've slipped down and I'm uncomfortable. (Sighs.)

Miss N: "There. Is that better?" (2)

Mr. H: "Yes, You're good to an old, tired, sick man."

Miss N: "Oh, you're not old, Mr. Holmes!" (3)

Mrs. H: "I feel it, my dear, I really do. (Sigh) Sometimes, I wonder if it's worth it."

Miss N: "What do you mean, Mr. Holmes?" (4)

Mr. H: "I hate being crippled up! I hate coming to the hospital, having tests, getting all riled up and for what? Just so they can tell me my arthritis is worse—or better—or the same. *I* can tell that, just by the way I feel! I don't need their fancy tests!"

Miss N: "They're always discovering new medicines, though. You shouldn't give up hope!" (5)

Mr. H: "What do I want with new medicines? In 5 more years I'll be dead anyway!"

Miss N: "You sound discouraged." (6)

Mr. H: "I am! I'm using part of my savings, coming in here 3 and 4 times a year. I don't get any better, and I won't! *They* know that! *I* know that! I'd rather be home with my wife and working in my wood shop when I can, waiting to die."

Miss N: "What do you make in your wood shop?" (7)

Mr. H: "Duck decoys! Leastways, I used to! Only made 3 last year 'cause my hands were so crippled up. I could have made 25 if I'd been able. People around here know I do good work."

Miss N: "You sound as though you'd like to be back home." (8)

Mr. H: "That's what I said, my dear! (Clears throat) I think I'll talk with some of them young doctors. Maybe they'll let me go, now that they got my medicine figured out again."

Miss N: "So you'd like to talk to them about it." (9)

Mr. H: "Yes, that's just what I'll do! Thanks for fixing my pillows."

YOUR ANSWER

1.

2.

3.

4.

5.

6.

7.

8.

9.

CORRECT ANSWER

1. Useful
2. Useful
3. a. Not useful
   b. "That is how you think of yourself?"
4. Useful
5. a. Not useful
   b. "You feel it's a waste of time coming to the hospital."
6. Useful
7. a. Not useful
   b. "You'd rather be home."
8. Useful
9. Useful

Appendix A

RESOURCE MATERIALS FOR THE PROGRAM

Glossary

A few technical terms used in the program are defined here for your convenience.

$\bar{a}$ — Before

ad lib   — As desired

↑ ad lib   — Ambulatory, up as desired

b.i.d.   — Twice a day

BRP   — Bathroom privileges (patient may get out of bed only to go to the bathroom)

$\bar{c}$ — With

E.C.   — Enteric-Coated

I. & O.   — Intake and output of liquids

IM   — Intramuscular (specifies route for medications)

IV   — Intravenous (specifies route for medications)

NPO   — Nothing by mouth

o   — Oral (specifies route for medications)

$\bar{p}$ — After

p.r.n.   — According to necessity (used in reference to medications which may be given if necessary with specified frequency)

P.T.   — Physical therapy

q.   — Every

q.d.   — Every day

q.h.   — Every hour

q.i.d.   — Four times a day

q.o.d.   — Every other day

q. 2°   — Every two hours

ROM   — Range of motion (movement of part of joint through its complete range)

$\bar{s}$ — Without

SCB   — Strictly confined to bed

t.i.d.   — Three times a day

TPR   — Temperature, pulse, and respiration

VS   — Vital signs (blood pressure, respiration, and pulse)

WA   — When awake

APPOINTMENT SCHEDULE

ON CALL _____ | _____

TIME	PATIENT Last Name, First Initial	APPOINTMENT	PATIENT Last Name, First Initial	APPOINTMENT
7:30				
8:00				
8:15				
8:30	Holmes, R	Physical Therapy		
8:45				
9:00				
9:15				
9:30	Willoughby, H	Portable Chest X-RAY		
9:45				
10:00				
10:15	Fulton, N.	AT bedside Chest X-RAY		
10:30				
10:45				
11:00	Groom, B	M3101 Kidney Function STUDIES		
11:15				

DATE _____   UNIT_____

LOCATION	NAME		SERVICE	AGE
5	Groom, Betty		Urology	37

EXP. DATE	STANDING MEDICATIONS	EXP. DATE	P. R. N. MEDICATIONS
2-12	Librium 10 mgm. (o) t.i.d. (10-2-6)	2-12	Compazine 10 mgm. (IM) q.4-6° prn nausea

ACME VISIBLE RECORDS VIRGINIA #84598-6

PRIVILEGES AND PRECAUTIONS:	TREATMENTS:
	Special skin care: Cleanse carefully
S.C.B.	and rub c̄ Dermassage lotion b.i.d.
	Special mouth care q̄ 2°:
I & O	½ H_2O_2 : ½ H_2O
Restrict fluids	
to 800 cc/day	
(including meals)	
	NPO p̄ midnight for kidney function studies
TPR q.4°	
VS q̄ 2°	
wt. q.d. (table)	

UNIVERSITY HOSPITAL - UNIVERSITY OF MICHIGAN

FORM 206007 4/63 10M REV. 6-59   NURSING CARE CARD

GUIDES TO NURSING MANAGEMENT:

1. Pt. doesn't like hospital soap because it dries her skin; has her own in her drawer.

2. Special mouth care: Pt. understands this and can do it if the equipment is provided. Besides $\frac{1}{2} H_2O_2 : \frac{1}{2} H_2O$, have pt brush teeth at least $\bar{p}$ every meal.

OPERATION AND DATE

DIAGNOSIS uremia -

DIET 40 gm. protein.   RELIGION Prot   ADMITTING DATE 4 days ago

LOCATION 5   NAME Groom, Betty   SERVICE Urology   AGE 37

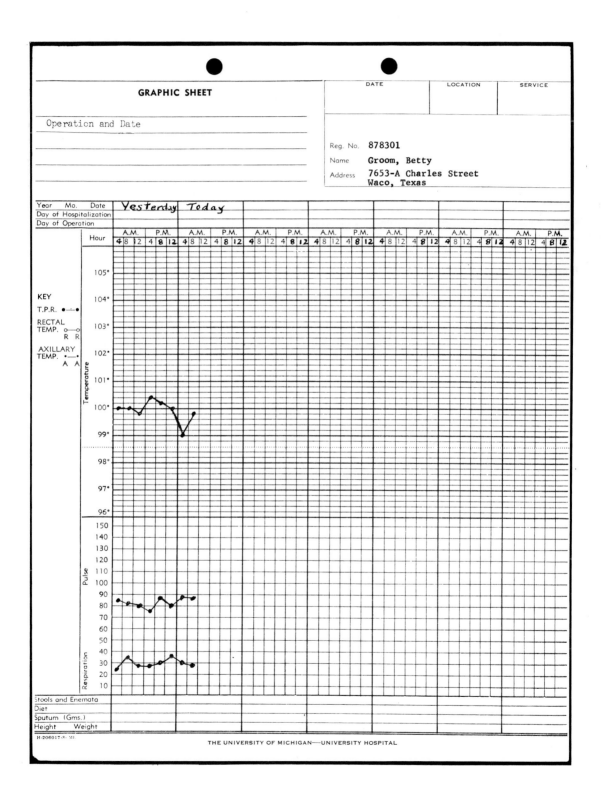

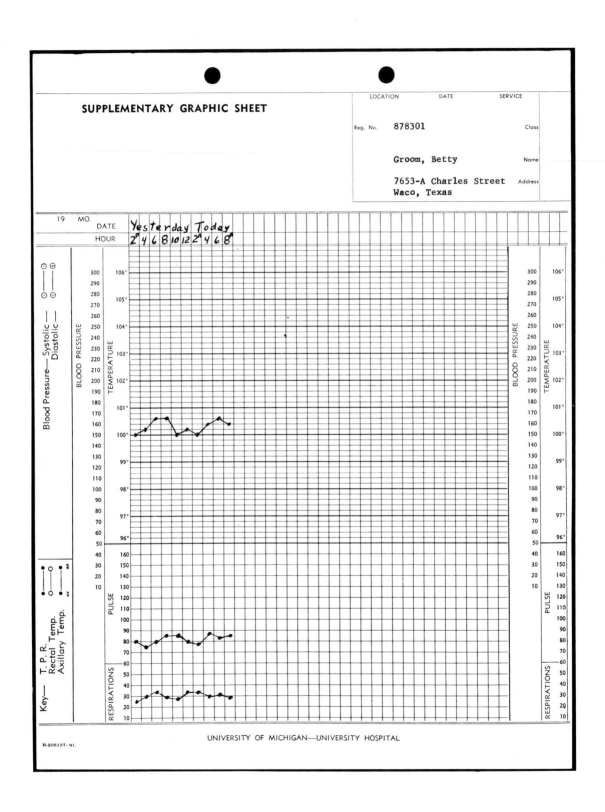

INTAKE AND OUTPUT

TOTAL SHEET

		LOCATION	DATE		SERVICE
Reg. No.	878301				Class
	Groom, Betty				Name
	7653-A Charles Street				Address
	Waco, Texas				

YR, MO. DATE	Yesterday			Today								
DAY OF HOSP.												
DAY OF OPERATION												
	8 A.M. 4 P.M.	4 P.M. 12 A.M.	12 A.M. 8 A.M.	8 A.M. 4 P.M.	4 P.M. 12 A.M.	12 A.M. 8 A.M.	8 A.M. 4 P.M.	4 P.M. 12 A.M.	12 A.M. 8 A.M.	8 A.M. 4 P.M.	4 P.M. 12 A.M.	12 A.M. 8 A.M.
INTAKE												
ORAL												
FORMULA												
INTRAVENOUS												
8 HOUR TOTAL	315	285	160									
24 HOUR TOTAL	xxxxxxxxxxxxxx	760cc	xxxxxxxxxxxxxx		xxxxxxxxxxxxx		xxxxxxxxxxxx					
OUTPUT												
URINARY												
8 HOUR TOTAL	60	200	45									
24 HOUR TOTAL	xxxxxxxxxxxxxx	305cc	xxxxxxxxxxxxxx		xxxxxxxxxxxxx		xxxxxxxxxxxx					
NON-URINARY												
EMESIS												
WANGENSTEEN												
BILE												
THORACOTOMY												
8 HOUR TOTAL												
24 HOUR TOTAL	xxxxxxxxxxxxxx		xxxxxxxxxxxxxx		xxxxxxxxxxxxx		xxxxxxxxxxxx					

H-206063-ML

THE UNIVERSITY OF MICHIGAN—UNIVERSITY HOSPITAL

MEDICATION RECORD

1. Routine medications – begin at top of sheet.
2. P.R.N. and stat medications and infusions – begin at bottom of sheet. Record all infusion solutions and added medications.
3. Medications given – write hour in appropriate column.
4. Medications omitted – write hour in appropriate column and circle hour. Note reason on blue notes.
5. Medications discontinued – write "Discontinued" following time of last dosage given.
6. Changes in orders – discontinue first order.
7. Sign full name for each tour of duty.

LOCATION   DATE   SERVICE

REG. NO.   878301   CLASS

NAME

Groom, Betty

ADDRESS

7653-A Charles. St.
Waco, Texas

MEDICATION ORDER	DATE Yesterday		DATE Today		DATE		FOR PHARMACY USE ONLY
	HOUR GIVEN		HOUR GIVEN		HOUR GIVEN		
DRUG DOSAGE ROUTE FREQ.	AM	PM	AM	PM	AM	PM	
Librium 10 mgm (o) t.i.d	10	2 6					
Compazine 10 mgm (IM)		6$\frac{30}{}$					
q 4-6° prn nausea							
	12:05 — 8:05	4:35 — 12:05	12:05 — 8:05	4:35 — 12:05	12:05 — 8:05	4:35 — 12:05	
SIGNATURE		C. Rucks	T. O'Neil				
	8:05 — 1:05	1:05 — 4:35	8:05 — 1:05	1:05 — 4:35	8:05 — 1:05	1:05 — 4:35	
		L. Ross					

H206189   THE UNIVERSITY OF MICHIGAN – UNIVERSITY HOSPITAL

BLUE COPY – MEDICAL RECORD

NURSING NOTES

1. Routines of care—write treatments and frequency; fill in time upon completion.
2. P.R.N. routines—write treatments and frequency, fill in time upon completion.
3. Write "AM" and "PM" midnite and noon only.
4. Leave two lines between routines and observations.
5. Write special tests or treatments and time completed above observations.
6. Write observations across full line.
7. Sign full name for each tour of duty.

LOCATION	DATE	SERVICE
Reg. No. 878301		Class

Groom, Betty   Name

7653-A Charles St. Address
Waco, Texas

HOUR	OBSERVATION	TREATMENT
		Yesterday
		Special mouth care $\bar{c}$ ½ H_2O_2 : ½ H_2O q 2°
		8/LR 10/LR 12/LR 2/LR 4/LR 6/CR 8/CR
		10/CR 12/CR
		Special skin care 10/LR 6/CR
8-4		Pt. has erythematous area the size of a quarter on her sacrum. Heat lamp applied for 20" – area less erythematous. Resting comfortably – afebrile. L. Ross
4-12		Pt. said she felt nauseated $\bar{p}$ supper. Compazine given $\bar{c}$ some relief. Heat lamp for 20" to erythematous area on sacrum. Appeared tired – said she wanted to sleep at 8³⁰. C. Ricts
		Today
12-8		NPO $\bar{p}$ midnight for kidney function studies. Slept fitfully. Awake at intervals. At 3ᴬᴹ appeared confused – sat up in bed and said, "Is dinner ready?" Did not know where she was. Calmed down in a few minutes and returned to sleep. Awoke again at 4³⁰ AM and was oriented as to place and time. VS stable. Skin dry and flaty – lotion applied. T. O'Neil

H-206025

THE UNIVERSITY OF MICHIGAN—UNIVERSITY HOSPITAL

LOCATION	NAME	SERVICE	AGE
14	Willoughby, Harold	Tho. Surg.	45

EXP. DATE	STANDING MEDICATIONS	EXP. DATE	P.R.N. MEDICATIONS
2-7	Procaine penicillin 400,000u IM b.i.d. (10-10)	2-7	Demerol 75 mgm. IM q 3-4° prn pain

#84598-6

PRIVILEGES AND PRECAUTIONS:	TREATMENTS:
chair T.I.D. for 30" May not lie on ℞ side	Chest tubes to bubble suction Cough & turn q 2° deep breathe q 2°
I+O encourage fluids to 3000 cc	R.O.M. to R arm and shoulder T.I.D.
TPR q. 4° VS. q.i.d.	

UNIVERSITY HOSPITAL - UNIVERSITY OF MICHIGAN

FORM 206007 4/63 10M REV. 6-59   NURSING CARE CARD

GUIDES TO NURSING MANAGEMENT:

1. Pt. finds coughing painful and resists doing it. Is more cooperative when nurse holds bath blanket around pt's chest to hold incision together.

2. Pt. likes grape and apple juice - dislikes citrus juices.

OPERATION AND DATE _Right lobectomy 4 days ago._

DIAGNOSIS _Cancer rt. lung_

DIET _Soft_

RELIGION _Cath_

ADMITTING DATE _1 week ago_

LOCATION _14_   NAME _Willoughby, Harold_

SERVICE _Thoracic Surg._   AGE _45_

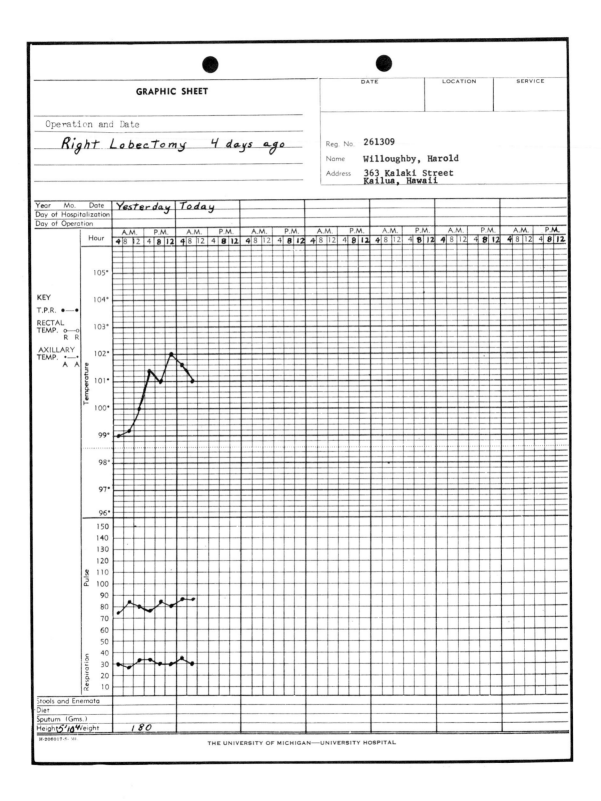

GRAPHIC SHEET

| DATE | LOCATION | SERVICE |

Operation and Date

Right Lobectomy   4 days ago

Reg. No. 261309

Name Willoughby, Harold

Address 363 Kalaki Street
Kailua, Hawaii

KEY

T.P.R. ●—●

RECTAL
TEMP. o—o
R   R

AXILLARY
TEMP. ●—·
A   A

Height 5'10" Weight   180

H-206017-8-5(1)

THE UNIVERSITY OF MICHIGAN—UNIVERSITY HOSPITAL

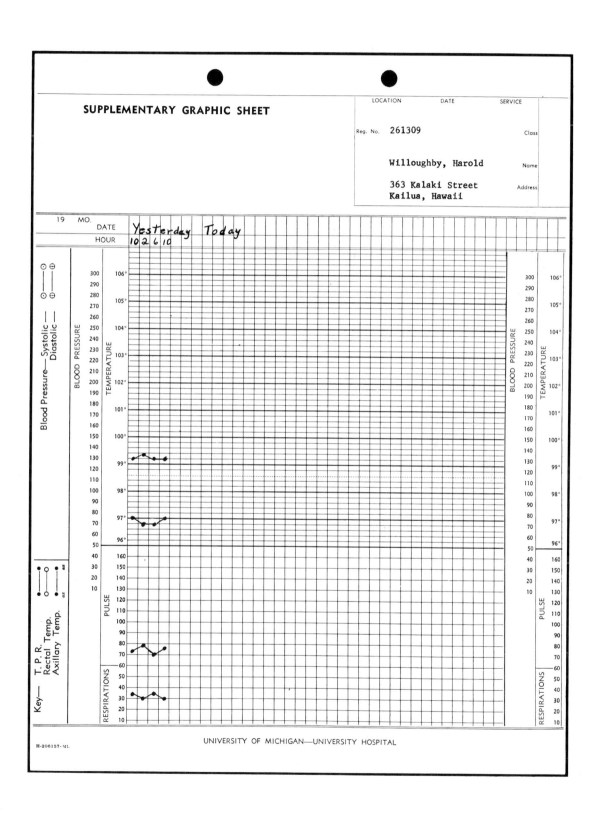

SUPPLEMENTARY GRAPHIC SHEET

LOCATION   DATE   SERVICE

Reg. No.   261309   Class

Willoughby, Harold   Name

363 Kalaki Street   Address
Kailua, Hawaii

H-206157-ML   UNIVERSITY OF MICHIGAN—UNIVERSITY HOSPITAL

INTAKE AND OUTPUT

TOTAL SHEET

LOCATION   DATE   SERVICE

Reg. No.   261309   Class

Willoughby, Harold   Name

363 Kalaki Street   Address
Kailua, Hawaii

YR, MO. DATE	Yesterday			Today								
DAY OF HOSP.												
DAY OF OPERATION												
	8 A.M. 4 P.M.	4 P.M. 12 A.M.	12 A.M. 8 A.M.	8 A.M. 4 P.M.	4 P.M. 12 A.M.	12 A.M. 8 A.M.	8 A.M. 4 P.M.	4 P.M. 12 A.M.	12 A.M. 8 A.M.	8 A.M. 4 P.M.	4 P.M. 12 A.M.	12 A.M. 8 A.M.

INTAKE

ORAL

FORMULA

INTRAVENOUS

8 HOUR TOTAL	1820	1440	200									
24 HOUR TOTAL	xxxxxxxxxxxxx	3460cc	xxxxxxxxxxxxx		xxxxxxxxxxxxx		xxxxxxxxxxxxx					

OUTPUT

URINARY

8 HOUR TOTAL	600	700	575									
24 HOUR TOTAL	xxxxxxxxxxxxx	1875cc	xxxxxxxxxxxxx		xxxxxxxxxxxxx		xxxxxxxxxxxxx					

NON-URINARY

EMESIS

WANGENSTEEN

BILE

THORACOTOMY

8 HOUR TOTAL	20cc	30cc	0									
24 HOUR TOTAL	xxxxxxxxxxxxx	50cc	xxxxxxxxxxxxx		xxxxxxxxxxxxx		xxxxxxxxxxxxx					

H-206063-ML   THE UNIVERSITY OF MICHIGAN—UNIVERSITY HOSPITAL

MEDICATION RECORD

1. Routine medications—begin at top of sheet.
2. P.R.N. and stat medications and infusions—begin at bottom of sheet. Record all infusion solutions and added medications.
3. Medications given—write hour in appropriate column.
4. Medications omitted—write hour in appropriate column and circle hour. Note reason on blue notes.
5. Medications discontinued—write "Discontinued" following time of last dosage given.
6. Changes in orders—discontinue first order.
7. Sign full name for each tour of duty.

LOCATION   DATE   SERVICE

REG. NO. **261309**   CLASS

Willoughby, Harold   NAME

363 Kalaki Street   ADDRESS
Kailua, Hawaii

MEDICATION ORDER	DATE Yesterday		DATE Today		DATE		FOR PHARMACY USE ONLY
	HOUR GIVEN		HOUR GIVEN		HOUR GIVEN		
DRUG DOSAGE ROUTE FREQ.	AM	PM	AM	PM	AM	PM	
Procaine Penicillin 400,000 U (IM) b.i.d.	10	10					
Demerol 75 mgm (IM) q3-4° p.r.n.		7^{30}					

SIGNATURE	12:05 — 8:05	4:35 — 12:05	12:05 — 8:05	4:35 — 12:05	12:05 — 8:05	4:35 — 12:05	
		C. Ricks	T. O'Neil				
	8:05 — 1:05	1:05 — 4:35	8:05 — 1:05	1:05 — 4:35	8:05 — 1:05	1:05 — 4:35	
		L. Ross					

H206189

THE UNIVERSITY OF MICHIGAN—UNIVERSITY HOSPITAL

BLUE COPY — MEDICAL RECORD

NURSING NOTES

1. Routines of care—write treatments and frequency; fill in time upon completion.
2. P.R.N. routines—write treatments and frequency, fill in time upon completion.
3. Write "AM" and "PM" midnite and noon only.
4. Leave two lines between routines and observations.
5. Write special tests or treatments and time completed above observations.
6. Write observations across full line.
7. Sign full name for each tour of duty.

LOCATION	DATE	SERVICE
Reg. No. 261309		Class

Willoughby, Harold — Name

363 Kalaki Street — Address
Kailua, Hawaii

HOUR	OBSERVATION	TREATMENT
		Yesterday
		ROM to (R) arm and shoulder t.i.d. 10/LR 2/LR 6/LR
		chair for 30" t.i.d. 10/LR 2/LR 6/LR
8-4		Small amt. of light red drainage through chest tubes. Pt. cough q 2° - productive of moderate amt. of thick white mucus. Up in chair twice c̄ no ill effects. Drinking fluids well. Says he is eager for the weekend to come so he can see his children. L. Ross
4-12		Quiet evening. After sitting in chair for 15", said he was tired and returned to bed. Appears diaphoretic. Cough is productive of moderate amt of thick whitish-green mucus. Requested med. for pain in (R) shoulder and operative site: given at 7:30 c̄ relief. Moves (R) arm well through range of motion. Since 8^{AM} drainage through chest tubes ± 50 cc light red. Dressing over incision is dry. C. Ricks
		Today
12-8		Slept fairly well. Coughing q 2° - productive of moderate amt of thick whitish green mucus. No more drainage through chest tubes during the night. Dressing remains dry. T. O'Neil

H-206025   THE UNIVERSITY OF MICHIGAN—UNIVERSITY HOSPITAL

LOCATION	NAME		SERVICE	AGE
10	Holmes, Robert		Medicine	75

EXP. DATE	STANDING MEDICATIONS	EXP. DATE	P.R.N. MEDICATIONS
2-20	Buffered ASA gr. x (o) q.i.d. (10-2-6-10)	2-20	Milk of Magnesia 30cc (o) prn constipation
2-20	Prednisone 2.5 mgm. (o) t.i.d. (10-2-6)	2-20	Darvon 65 mgm (o) p.r.n pain
2-20	Diuril 0.5 gm. (o) b.i.d (10-6)		
2-20	EC KCl 1.0 gm. (o) b.i.d. (10-6)		

ACME VISIBLE #84598-6

PRIVILEGES AND PRECAUTIONS:	TREATMENTS:
ambulate pt.	Heating pad to rt. shoulder for 30" q.i.d.
the length of the	ROM to all extremities at least b.i.d
hall at least tid	
110	
	early breakfast
TPR q.i.d.	P.T. at. 8:30 A.M.
wt q.o.d. (odd)	

UNIVERSITY HOSPITAL - UNIVERSITY OF MICHIGAN

FORM 206007 4/63 10M REV. 6-59   NURSING CARE CARD

GUIDES TO NURSING MANAGEMENT:

1. Pt. prefers 2 pillows behind his back and one between his knees and lower legs when lying on his right side.

2. ROM to all extremities is carried out $\bar{c}$ less fatigue to pt. if done immed. $\bar{p}$ breakfast & $\bar{p}$ supper.

3. Pt. understands importance of ROM & can do his upper extremities but needs help $\bar{c}$ his lower ones.

OPERATION AND DATE

DIAGNOSIS   Rheumatoid arthritis.

DIET   No added salt.

RELIGION   Pres

ADMITTING DATE   1 wk. ago

LOCATION   10

NAME   HOLMES. RoberT

SERVICE   Med.

AGE   75

GRAPHIC SHEET

	DATE	LOCATION	SERVICE

Operation and Date

Reg. No. **822606**

Name **Holmes, Robert**

Address **9123 Webb Street**
Tecumseh, Michigan

Year Mo. Date													
Day of Hospitalization													
Day of Operation													

KEY

T.P.R. ●—●

RECTAL
TEMP. o—o
    R R

AXILLARY
TEMP. ·—·
    A A

Temperature scale: 105°, 104°, 103°, 102°, 101°, 100°, 99°, 98°, 97°, 96°

Pulse scale: 150, 140, 130, 120, 110, 100, 90, 80, 70, 60, 50, 40, 30, 20, 10

Respiration

Stools and Enemata													
Diet													
Sputum (Gms.)													
Height 5'9 Weight	155												

H-206017-S-MI

THE UNIVERSITY OF MICHIGAN—UNIVERSITY HOSPITAL

	LOCATION	DATE	SERVICE
Reg. No.	822606		Class
	Holmes, Robert		Name
	9123 Webb Street		Address
	Tecumseh, Michigan		

INTAKE AND OUTPUT

TOTAL SHEET

	Yesterday			Today								
YR. MO. DATE / DAY OF HOSP. / DAY OF OPERATION	8 A.M. 4 P.M.	4 P.M. 12 A.M.	12 A.M. 8 A.M.	8 A.M. 4 P.M.	4 P.M. 12 A.M.	12 A.M. 8 A.M.	8 A.M. 4 P.M.	4 P.M. 12 A.M.	12 A.M. 8 A.M.	8 A.M. 4 P.M.	4 P.M. 12 A.M.	12 A.M. 8 A.M.
INTAKE												
ORAL												
FORMULA												
INTRAVENOUS												
8 HOUR TOTAL	1100	950	300									
24 HOUR TOTAL	xxxxxxxxxxxxxx	2350cc		xxxxxxxxxxxxxx			xxxxxxxxxxxxx			xxxxxxxxxxxxx		
OUTPUT												
URINARY												
8 HOUR TOTAL	800	525	375									
24 HOUR TOTAL	xxxxxxxxxxxxxx	1700cc		xxxxxxxxxxxxxx			xxxxxxxxxxxxx			xxxxxxxxxxxxx		
NON-URINARY												
EMESIS												
WANGENSTEEN												
BILE												
THORACOTOMY												
8 HOUR TOTAL												
24 HOUR TOTAL	xxxxxxxxxxxxxx			xxxxxxxxxxxxxx			xxxxxxxxxxxxxx			xxxxxxxxxxxxx		

H-206063-ML

THE UNIVERSITY OF MICHIGAN—UNIVERSITY HOSPITAL

MEDICATION RECORD

1. Routine medications—begin at top of sheet.
2. P.R.N. and stat medications and infusions—begin at bottom of sheet. Record all infusion solutions and added medications.
3. Medications given—write hour in appropriate column.
4. Medications omitted—write hour in appropriate column and circle hour. Note reason on blue notes.
5. Medications discontinued—write "Discontinued" following time of last dosage given.
6. Changes in orders—discontinue first order.
7. Sign full name for each tour of duty.

LOCATION   DATE   SERVICE

REG. NO.   822606   CLASS

NAME   Holmes, Robert

ADDRESS   9123 Webb Street
Tecumseh, Michigan

MEDICATION ORDER	DATE Yesterday		DATE Today		DATE		FOR PHARMACY USE ONLY	
	HOUR GIVEN		HOUR GIVEN		HOUR GIVEN			
DRUG DOSAGE ROUTE FREQ.	AM	PM	AM	PM	AM	PM		
Buffered ASA gr X (o) q.i.d	10	2 6 10						
Prednisone 2.5 mgm (o) t.i.d	10	2 6						
Diuril 0.5 gm. (O) b.i.d.	10	6						
E.C. KCL 1.0 gm. (O) b.i.d.	10	6						
Darvon 65 mgm (o) p.r.n. pain		9³⁰						
SIGNATURE	12:05 — 8:05	4:35 — 12:05 C. Ricks	12:05 — 8:05 T. O'Neil	4:35 — 12:05	12:05 — 8:05	4:35 — 12:05		
	8:05 — 1:05 L. Ross	1:05 — 4:35	8:05 — 1:05	1:05 — 4:35	8:05 — 1:05	1:05 — 4:35		

H206189   THE UNIVERSITY OF MICHIGAN—UNIVERSITY HOSPITAL

BLUE COPY — MEDICAL RECORD

NURSING NOTES

1. Routines of care—write treatments and frequency; fill in time upon completion.
2. P.R.N. routines—write treatments and frequency, fill in time upon completion.
3. Write "AM" and "PM" midnite and noon only.
4. Leave two lines between routines and observations.
5. Write special tests or treatments and time completed above observations.
6. Write observations across full line.
7. Sign full name for each tour of duty.

LOCATION	DATE	SERVICE
Reg. No.	822606	Class

Name
Holmes, Robert
9123 Webb Street
Tecumseh, Michigan   Address

HOUR	OBSERVATION	TREATMENT
		Yesterday
		Heating pad to (R) shoulder for 30" q.i.d. 10/L.R. 2/L.R. 4/C.R. 10/C.R.
		ROM to all extremities b.i.d. 10/L.P. 7/C.R.
		Ambulate t.i.d. 10/L.R. 2/L.R. 6/C.R.
8-4		To PT at 8:30. Walked the length of the hall when he returned. Says that he thinks his right shoulder is less painful today. L. Ross
4-12		Walked out to ward to visit another pt. Requested medication for pain in (R) shoulder. Given at 9:30 c̄ relief. C. Ricks
		Today
12-8		Slept well T. O'Neil

Verbal Report from Night Nurse to Day Nurse: 8:00 A.M.

"Mr. Holmes slept very well last night. He had Darvon 65 mgm. for pain in his right shoulder at 9:30 last night and hasn't asked for anything since. His TPR this morning is 99^6, 74, and 26. His oral intake from 8:00 A.M. yesterday until 8:00 A.M. today was 2350 cc., output was 1700 cc. He had an early breakfast so he'll be ready for his P.T. appointment at 8:30 A.M."

LOCATION	NAME		SERVICE	AGE
17	FulTon Nora		Allergy	33

EXP. DATE	STANDING MEDICATIONS	EXP. DATE	P. R. N. MEDICATIONS
5-21	multivits cap. I (o) q. 1 (10)	5/21	Aminophylline suppositor
5-21	Elixir terpin hydrate 1 tsp. (o) q. 4° (10-2-6 etc.)		I (R) q. 12° p.r.n. dyspnea.
5-21	Tetracycline hydrochloride 250 mgm. (o) q. 6° (10-4-10-4)		

ACME VISIBLE RECORDS VIRGINIA #84598-6

PRIVILEGES AND PRECAUTIONS:	TREATMENTS:
↑ ad lib	Postural drainage for 15" t.i.d ā meals Cough q. 2° while awake
I & O	
Encourage fluids at least 1C. phr	
TPR q 4°	

UNIVERSITY HOSPITAL - UNIVERSITY OF MICHIGAN

FORM 206007 4/63 10M REV. 6-59

NURSING CARE CARD

GUIDES TO NURSING MANAGEMENT:

1. Likes grape juice and pineapple juice

OPERATION AND DATE

DIAGNOSIS *Asthma* *?Pneumonia*

DIET *General*

| | | RELIGION *Ca* | ADMITTING DATE *Yesterday* |

| LOCATION 77 | NAME Fulton, Nora | | SERVICE *Allergy* | AGE 33 |

GRAPHIC SHEET

DATE	LOCATION	SERVICE

Operation and Date

Reg. No. 800606-4
Name Fulton, Nora (Mrs.)
Address 2341 Banbury Lane
Flint, Michigan

Year Mo. Date	Yesterday	Today					
Day of Hospitalization	1	2					
Day of Operation							

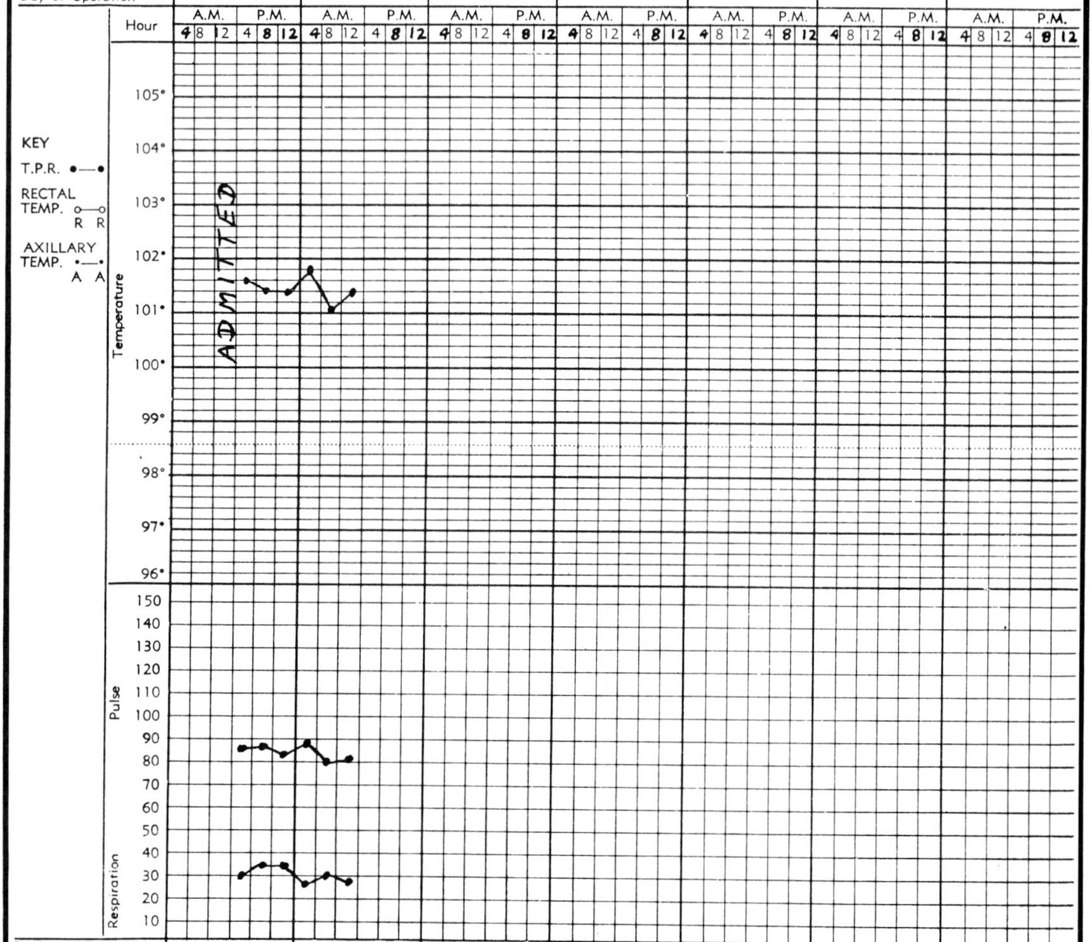

Hour
A.M. P.M.
4 8 12 4 8 12
KEY
T.P.R. •—•
RECTAL TEMP. o—o R R
AXILLARY TEMP. •-—• A A
Temperature
105° 104° 103° 102° 101° 100° 99° 98° 97° 96°
ADMITTED
Pulse
150 140 130 120 110 100 90 80 70 60 50
Respiration
40 30 20 10

Stools and Enemata							
Diet							
Sputum (Gms.)							
Height 5'5" Weight	126						

H-206017-S-MI

THE UNIVERSITY OF MICHIGAN—UNIVERSITY HOSPITAL

INTAKE AND OUTPUT

TOTAL SHEET

LOCATION	DATE	SERVICE
Reg. No. 800606-4		Class
Fulton, Nora (Mrs.)		Name
2341 Banbury Lane Flint, Michigan		Address

YR. MO. DATE	Yesterday			Today								
DAY OF HOSP.												
DAY OF OPERATION												
	8 A.M. 4 P.M.	4 P.M. 12 A.M.	12 A.M. 8 A.M.	8 A.M. 4 P.M.	4 P.M. 12 A.M.	12 A.M. 8 A.M.	8 A.M. 4 P.M.	4 P.M. 12 A.M.	12 A.M. 8 A.M.	8 A.M. 4 P.M.	4 P.M. 12 A.M.	12 A.M. 8 A.M.
INTAKE												
ORAL	220	650	210									
FORMULA												
INTRAVENOUS												
8 HOUR TOTAL												
24 HOUR TOTAL	xxxxxxxxxxxxx		1080	xxxxxxxxxxxxxx			xxxxxxxxxxxxx			xxxxxxxxxxxxx		
OUTPUT												
URINARY												
8 HOUR TOTAL		380	220									
24 HOUR TOTAL	xxxxxxxxxxxxx		600	xxxxxxxxxxxxxx			xxxxxxxxxxxxx			xxxxxxxxxxxxx		
NON-URINARY												
EMESIS												
WANGENSTEEN												
BILE												
THORACOTOMY												
8 HOUR TOTAL												
24 HOUR TOTAL	xxxxxxxxxxxxx			xxxxxxxxxxxxxx			xxxxxxxxxxxxx			xxxxxxxxxxxxx		

H-206063-ML   THE UNIVERSITY OF MICHIGAN—UNIVERSITY HOSPITAL

MEDICATION RECORD

1. Routine medications – begin at top of sheet.
2. P.R.N and stat medications and infusions – begin at bottom of sheet.
   Record all infusion solutions and added medications.
3. Medications given – write hour in appropriate column.
4. Medications omitted – write hour in appropriate column and circle
   hour. Note reason on blue notes.
5. Medications discontinued – write "Discontinued" following time of
   last dosage given.
6. Changes in orders – discontinue first order.
7. Sign full name for each tour of duty.

LOCATION	DATE	SERVICE

REG. NO.   800606-4   CLASS

Fulton, Nora (Mrs.)   NAME

2341 Banbury Lane   ADDRESS
Flint, Michigan

MEDICATION ORDER				DATE Yesterday		DATE Today		DATE		FOR PHARMACY USE ONLY
				HOUR GIVEN		HOUR GIVEN		HOUR GIVEN		
DRUG	DOSAGE	ROUTE	FREQ.	AM	PM	AM	PM	AM	PM	
Elixir Terpin hydrate /tsp (o) q 4°					2,6,10	2,6				
Tetracycline hydrachloride 250 mgm (o) q 6°					4,10	4				
Aminophylline suppository ī (B) q 12° prn dyspnea										

SIGNATURE	12:05 — 8:05	4:35 — 12:05 C. Ricko	12:05 — 8:05 T. O'Neil	4:35 — 12:05	12:05 — 8:05	4:35 — 12:05
	8:05 — 1:05	1:05 — 4:35 L. Ross	8:05 — 1:05	1:05 — 4:35	8:05 — 1:05	1:05 — 4:35

H206189   THE UNIVERSITY OF MICHIGAN – UNIVERSITY HOSPITAL

BLUE COPY – MEDICAL RECORD

NURSING NOTES

1. Routines of care—write treatments and frequency; fill in time upon completion.
2. P.R.N. routines—write treatments and frequency; fill in time upon completion.
3. Write "AM" and "PM" midnite and noon only.
4. Leave two lines between routines and observations.
5. Write special tests or treatments and time completed above observations.
6. Write observations across full line.
7. Sign full name for each tour of duty.

LOCATION	DATE	SERVICE
Reg. No. 800606-4		Class
Fulton, Nora (Mrs.)		Name
2341 Banbury Lane Flint, Michigan		Address

HOUR	OBSERVATION	TREATMENT

Yesterday

2 p.m. 33 year old woman admitted to ward, bed #17, via wheelchair. Pt. appears to be dyspneic at intervals. Temp. 101⁶, P 86, R 30. States that she is here because, "I can't catch my breath". Urine specimen obtained.

4 p.m. Pt. resting in bed c̄ head ↑ 45°, coughs productively: thick whitish-green mucus. Drinking fluids.   L. Ross

7 p.m. Pt. extremely dyspneic. Dr. notified. R 36 — shallow. Aminophylline suppository given.

7⁴³ Dr. Knowles here to see pt. Pt. breathing more easily. T 101⁴ P 98 R 30 — irregular.

8⁰⁰ Pt. continues to breathe easily. R 24 slightly irregular

12⁰⁰ Pt. having no dyspnea. Asleep c̄ bed in Semi-Fowler's position   C. Ricks

Today

3 a.m. Pt. awoke — appeared slightly dyspneic. P 96 R 30 Sat upright on edge of bed for a few minutes — then said she felt better. Breathing appeared less difficult. R 24 Slept most of the rest of the night.
                    T. O'Neil

H-206025   THE UNIVERSITY OF MICHIGAN—UNIVERSITY HOSPITAL

Verbal Report from Night Nurse to Day Nurse: 8:00 A.M.

"Mrs. Fulton is in 17. Her temperature is still elevated:
T 101°, P 80, and R 30. She was quite dyspneic last night
after supper. She had an aminophylline suppository and that
helped her to breathe easier. Dr. Knowles came over then and
said just keep an eye on her. She slept pretty well, her bed
was in semi-Fowler's position. She woke up once at 3:00 A.M.
and was slightly dyspneic, but then she just sat on the edge
of the bed and after a few minutes she was okay. Her oral
intake since she was admitted yesterday until 8:00 A.M. today
was 1080 cc.; output was 600 cc. She's to have a portable
chest x-ray at her bedside at 10:15 this morning."

Appendix B

CRITERION TEST

In these pages we will introduce you to Mr. James and Mrs. Wicker, two patients. You will be asked to respond in writing as you would respond orally to the patient, to seek information when necessary, and to act upon the information you have found. In order to make these situations as similar to the clinical situations as possible, we have provided supplementary material in which data are recorded as they are in the clinical area. All information is complete. Medical information pertinent to the patients is in Appendix C. Consult this information at any time you wish.

First answer all questions pertinent to Mr. James; then answer all questions pertinent to Mrs. Wicker. *When the test asks you what you would say to the patient, state the exact words you would use. When you are asked what action you would take or what you would do, describe your action in concrete terms.*

Remember that you will be in the clinical area from 8:00 A.M. until 12:00 noon. This is the first time you have cared for both patients.

Mr. James

J–1 You are assigned to care for Mr. Rudolph James. Look at his data booklet and write your answers to each of the following questions.

1. What is his diagnosis?

2. Does he have any appointments? If so, what? At what time? What preparation is necessary, if any?

3. Will I have to give him any medications this morning? What are they? What amount? What route? What frequency? What time?

4. Describe how he slept last night.

Now you are ready to enter the unit and see Mr. James for the first time.

J–2 You walk into Mr. James's unit at 8:15 A.M. The head of his bed is slightly elevated. His head is resting on two pillows; his hair is unruly. He is wearing hospital pajamas and is covered by a slightly wrinkled sheet. To his left is the overbed table and to his right is the bedside stand on which a water pitcher is placed. The unit as a whole appears to be neat.

Mr. James looks up as you enter and says, "Hello there, young lady!"

J–3 A few minutes later, at 8:25 A.M., you walk into the ward. You notice that all of the other men in the ward have their breakfast. Mr. James is reclining in bed with his overbed table in front of him. He points to the men on either side of him and then says to you:

"These two guys have been eating for ten minutes, and I'm getting awfully hungry! Aren't I going to have breakfast today?"

What would you say to Mr. James?

J–4 At 9:00 o'clock you come back to remove Mr. James' breakfast tray from his unit. As you near the bedside and are about to lift the tray from the overbed table, he says to you in a low, confidential tone, "You know, I was awake late last night watching TV, and that man over there (points to Mr. Cutler across the ward in bed 5) kept moaning and crying so that I could hardly hear the TV. I know he had his foot amputated two days ago, and he probably has some pain, but he's *really* carrying on! What's the matter with him, anyhow?"

You remember hearing about Mr. Cutler in morning report. (You may refer to the data in morning report to refresh your memory if you wish.)

What do you say to Mr. James?

J–5 At about 10:00 A.M. you take Mr. James's vital signs. They are 140/82, P. 70, and R. 28.

Is any action indicated beyond recording these figures in the patient's chart? Why or why not?

J–6 Now it is 10:30 A.M. and Mr. James has had his electrocardiogram and his bath. You begin to make his bed while he is sitting up in the chair in the unit. After several minutes of comfortable silence, Mr. James remarks, "You seem awfully young to be a nurse. Whatever made you decide to become a nurse?"

What do you say to Mr. James?

J–7 As Mr. James is sitting in the chair, a magazine slides from his lap to the floor. As he leans over to retrieve it, he exclaims, "Ooh! My back *really* hurts!"

How would you respond?

J–8 As you continue to talk with Mr. James about his painful back, he says, "Well, he told me that if I moved quickly I might feel a sharp pain in my back for a short time." How would you respond?

J–9 Mr. James has been sitting up in the chair for twenty minutes. You have finished with the bed. You turn to him and say,

J–10 Mr. James returns to bed and lies on his left side with his head pillowed on his bent arm. He appears to be lost in thought, staring at a spot on the opposite wall. You adjust the covers and position a pillow comfortably behind his back. As you finish he rouses from thought, looks at you, and says, "I know there's something wrong with my heart, but there are a lot of things I'm still uncertain about. I wonder if you could answer some questions for me about my diagnosis?"

How do you respond?

J–11 A few minutes later he looks down at the bed covers and begins to slowly smooth them with is right hand. "Well," he says slowly, "I feel very depressed about my heart condition."

How do you respond?

J–12 Your conversation with Mr. James continues. State whether each of the nurse's responses, numbered 1 through 7, is useful or not useful. If her response is not useful, suggest a better one.

Mr. James: "The future is so uncertain! Some people who have heart problems like mine do go back to work successfully, but others try it and just can't make it."
Nurse: "And you are wondering which you will do." (1)
Mr. James: "Yes. We have four young children. How can I provide for them if I can't work?" (Begins to rub his forehead with his left hand)
Nurse: "Then taking care of your family's financial needs is one of your major concerns?" (2)
Mr. James: "It sure is! It's on my mind all the time! My wife says not to worry about it now. That the most important thing to do now is concentrate on getting well. I know that!"
Nurse: "Uh-huh" (3)
Mr. James: "But, I've been in here so long—and I'm still so weak. Twenty minutes in that chair and I'm ready for bed again. When am I ever going to feel good again?"
Nurse: "Oh, you will, Mr. James, It just takes time." (4)
Mr. James: "But I've been here so long—a month already, and I'm still so weak."
Nurse: "You feel discouraged about your progress." (5)
Mr. James: "I sure do! (said somewhat bitterly!) All my life I've saved and waited—didn't get married till I had a good job. Then didn't have kids till I was moving up, being promoted—earning enough money to support them—then POW! Knocked flat by a heart attack! What's the use?"
Nurse: "How old are your children, Mr. James?" (6)
Mr. James: "They're young—all under eight . . . Well, I've talked enough about my family and my problems."
Nurse: "No—I am interested in you and your situation. You sound very discouraged about how things are going." (7)
Mr. James: "Yes, my progress has been too slow to suit me. I'm amazed at how weak I've become while in the hospital . . . ."

Useful?	*Not Useful?*	*Better Response?*

1.

2.

3.

4.

5.

6.

7.

J–13 It is 11:30 A.M. You have completed Mr. James' care. He appears to want to rest, and you feel that you have met all of his immediate needs. As you leave to do your charting, you say to Mr. James,

Mrs. Wicker

W–1 You are assigned to care for Mrs. Gloria Wicker. Look at her data booklet and write your answers to each of the following questions.

1. What is her diagnosis?

2. What treatments does she have today? How many times a day should each treatment be done? For how long?

3. Is her temperature elevated?

4. Has she had any pain medication since last evening? What was it? How much? At what time?

Now suppose that during the morning Mrs. Wicker makes the following comments or asks you the following questions. In the space to the right of each question put your response *(verbatim)*.

Question	*Response (verbatim)*
5. "I'm so hungry; this breakfast isn't enough. Would you get me another donut and a glass of milk?"	5.
6. "I think I'll slip into my robe and go visit Mrs. Carter down the hall."	6.
7. "Oh, let me just sit here with my feet over the side of the bed while you wash my back."	7.

W–2 Look again at Mrs. Wicker's kardex and night report. Then write below four initial things you want to find out.

Now you are ready to enter the unit and see Mrs. Wicker for the first time.

W–3 You enter Mrs. Wicker's unit at 8:15 A.M. and find her curled up in the center of her bed crying and making low moaning sounds. Her bed covers and pajamas are extremely wrinkled; she is perspiring and her hair is unruly and wet around her face and neck. Three empty used glasses are on the overbed table to her left. Some juice has spilled around them. There are several get well cards on her bedside stand as well as a vase of flowers with drooping petals.

There are several wadded Kleenex lying on her bed and strewn on the floor and the bedside stand. The window shade is lowered, and the unit is in semi-darkness.

You hesitate a moment at the foot of the bed, cough softly, and then say:

W–4 You have straightened Mrs. Wicker's covers and helped her wash her face. You have cleaned up her unit, disposing of the used Kleenex and carrying out the dirty glasses. You have also raised the window shade part way. Mrs. Wicker has stopped crying, and the conversation continues. She says, "I wish I didn't have to keep my leg on these pillows all the time. It gets uncomfortable in the same position. Why do I have to keep it up on the pillows?"

Write down what you would say to Mrs. Wicker.

W–5 You have left to obtain Mrs. Wicker's bathing supplies. As you return to her bedside, she is talking with another nurse. You overhear the following conversation. State whether each of the nurse's responses, numbered 1 through 5, is useful or not useful. If the nurse's response is not useful, suggest a better one.

Mrs. Wicker: "Do you know, when I was talking to the Doctor, he told me that I might have to have my leg amputated!"

Nurse: "Tell me more about what he said." (1)

Mrs. Wicker: "He says that if it doesn't heal, I may be in real trouble because the sore is open nearly to the bone. He says that I just can't go on having an open sore like that, because it is easily infected and if the bone gets infected, that could be very bad. It frightens me to think of having a bone infection."

Nurse: "Generally—one can tell within a couple of weeks how the healing is progressing." (2)

Mrs. Wicker: "Well, there are worse things than having your leg amputated. I have lived with constant pain in my ankle for over a year now. Sometimes I think I'd be better off to have the amputation and get rid of the pain and constant medication. What do you think?"

Nurse: "I would never have an amputation! They are always coming up with new medicines and they might find one that would cure your sore." (3)

Mrs. Wicker: "Perhaps. But who knows how far in the future that would be. I need relief from the pain now!"

Nurse: "You don't look too comfortable with those pillows all crunched up under your leg; let me change them around." (4)

Mrs. Wicker: "That wasn't really necessary. I just need some time to think about this decision—and of course, time to see if my sore will heal.

Nurse: "I have to leave now, Mrs. Wicker. The student here is ready to give you your bath." (5)

  Useful?   *Not Useful?*   *Better Response?*

  1.

  2.

  3.

  4.

  5.

W–6 It is 9:15 A.M. You have the curtains drawn around Mrs. Wicker's unit. For the past hour you have been giving her a bath. Now she is resting comfortably on her right side covered with the bath blanket. You have placed a pillow under her lower left leg, and are preparing to rub her back. The following conversation takes place.

Nurse: "Well, Mrs. Wicker, I'm ready to rub your back now. I have here some creamy lotion and some alcohol. Which would you prefer?"

Mrs. Wicker: "I like lotion better. That alcohol really dries out my skin. One nurse used some last night and didn't even ask me about it. My back itched all night."

Nurse: "Yes, lotion is less drying than alcohol." (Proceeds to rub Mrs. Wicker's back. A moment of comfortable silence passes.)

Mrs. Wicker: "You're the first nurse who has thought to pull that pillow under my lower leg and ankle when I'm on my side. It's so thoughtful of you, since it hurts when my left ankle rests on my right ankle. You wouldn't think that would bother anyone as fat as me, but it does! At home I have a little stool I use to prop my foot on, but here I have to prop it up against my other foot. It's such a strain doing that and then trying to keep the covers off of it, too!"

Nurse: "Oh . . ."

Mrs. Wicker: "You wouldn't think that something as light as the covers on that foot would make any difference but they just press on it enough to make my ankle begin to throb!"

Nurse: "You should have a little cradle to put over your left foot. The cradle is like a round cage that rests on the bed—you put your foot in it and the covers rest over it, off of your foot."

Mrs. Wicker: "That sounds wonderful! Hmm, look at that snow out there. Guess I won't have any visitors today!"

Nurse: "Do you live far from here?"

Mrs. Wicker: "Just in Saline, but that road is so curvy. I really worry about my husband driving on it in this weather."

Nurse: "You'd rather he stayed home, safe and sound?"

Mrs. Wicker: "Yes, I sure would! Even though he is a good driver."

Nurse: "Yes. I'm finished rubbing your back. Let me help you get dressed."

During this conversation you have received some information about Mrs. Wicker's preference in nursing care.

State below what information you received. To whom are you going to communicate this information, and where are you going to write it down?

YOU MAY REFER BACK TO THE ENTIRE CONVERSATION.

Information Received　　　　　　　　*Communicated and/or Written Action Taken*

W–7 It is 9:30 A.M. Mrs. Wicker is comfortably resting in bed. You know that soon it will be time for the sterile compress to her ulcer. You find out from her that she has never had a sterile compress before.

    What do you say to her?

W–8 Suppose that Mrs. Wicker clutches at her covers and says, "No, I don't want the compress! I'm afraid it will hurt!"

    What do you say to Mrs. Wicker?

W–9 Mrs. Wicker says, "Mrs. MacKenzie, over there in that bed, told me that the nurses bring in the compresses piping hot so they won't cool off so fast. She says she's been *burned* a couple of times! I don't want that to happen to me!"

    What do you say to her now?

W–10 Later in the morning Mrs. Wicker again begins to talk with you about her illness. She states, "I just don't think the foods in my diet are what I need."

    How would you respond?

W–11 The conversation continues.

Mrs. Wicker: "The food here all tastes the same—and looks the same! Grey roast beef—grey potatoes—grey beans! I just don't like it. I know that a diabetic diet doesn't have to be like that because the one I followed at home tasted good."

Nurse: "What kinds of food did you eat at home?"

Mrs. Wicker: "I ate a lot of salads and vegetables. Most of my protein comes from fish. Here, they give me so much heavy meat like lamb and beef."

Nurse: "You don't like to eat a lot of meat then."

Mrs. Wicker: "No, I believe that meat makes one's system sluggish and hinders the body's healing abilities. You know how important it is for diabetics to have healthy skin? Fresh vegetables and fish help you to keep you skin healthier. It worries me that I can't get those things here."

    How do you respond?

W–12 When the problem situation is clear to both you and Mrs. Wicker, what is your goal?

W–13 You have just taken Mrs. Wicker's noon TPR. It is T. 99^2 P. 72, and R. 24. She is resting comfortably in bed with the foot cradle over her elevated left foot. You feel that you have met all her immediate needs. You have terminated your conversation with her.

In the space below, chart Mrs. Wicker's warm compress as you would in the nursing notes on the chart.

Appendix C

RESOURCE MATERIALS FOR THE CRITERION TEST

Appointment Sheet

On Call _____ _____
_____|_____ _____

TIME	Patient Last Name	First Initial	APPOINTMENT	Patient Last Name	First Initial	APPOINTMENT
7:30						
8:00	Thompson,	D.	Cysto			
8:15	Jonesboro,	C.	UGI			
8:30	Blackburn,	C.	Portable Chest x-ray			
8:45	Burlington,	V.	bronchogram			
9:00						
9:15	Williams,	T.	Radiation Therapy			
9:30	Brown,	J.	EMG			
9:45						
10:00	James,	R.	At Bedside EKG			
10:15	Fulton,	N.	At Bedside Chest x-ray			
10:30	Witherspoon,	M.	EKG			
10:45						
11:00	Dickson,	R.	Radiation Therapy			
11:15						

DATE _____ UNIT _____

LOCATION	NAME		SERVICE	AGE
15	James, Rudolph		Medicine	43

EXP. DATE	STANDING MEDICATIONS	EXP. DATE	P.R.N. MEDICATIONS
3-16	Colace 100 mgm (o) q.d. (10ᴬ)	3-16	Darvon 65 mgm (o) q 4-6
3-16	Digitoxin 0.1 mgm (o) q.d.		prn headache
	(10ᴬ)	3-16	Seconal 100 mgm (o) h.s
			p.r.n May repeat x 1

ACME VISIBLE CROZET VIRGINIA #84598-6

PRIVILEGES AND PRECAUTIONS:	TREATMENTS:
Up in chair 20" t.i.d.	
1 & O	
VS b.i.d.	
wt. q.d.	

1. Have pt. void ear ½ hour prior to test.
2. Bathe pt. prior to test.

UNIVERSITY HOSPITAL - UNIVERSITY OF MICHIGAN
FORM 206007 4/63 10M REV. 6-59   NURSING CARE CARD

GUIDES TO NURSING MANAGEMENT:

1. Pt expresses concern about how his wife is
managing ⊤ their 4 small children (ages
2-7), even though he is receiving sick
pay from the factory where he works
as a foreman.

OPERATION AND DATE

DIAGNOSIS   Congestive Heart failure

DIET   Low sodium

	I	O	RELIGION	ADMITTING DATE
	✓	✓	Cath	1 month ago

LOCATION	NAME	SERVICE	AGE
15	James, Rudolph	Medicine	43

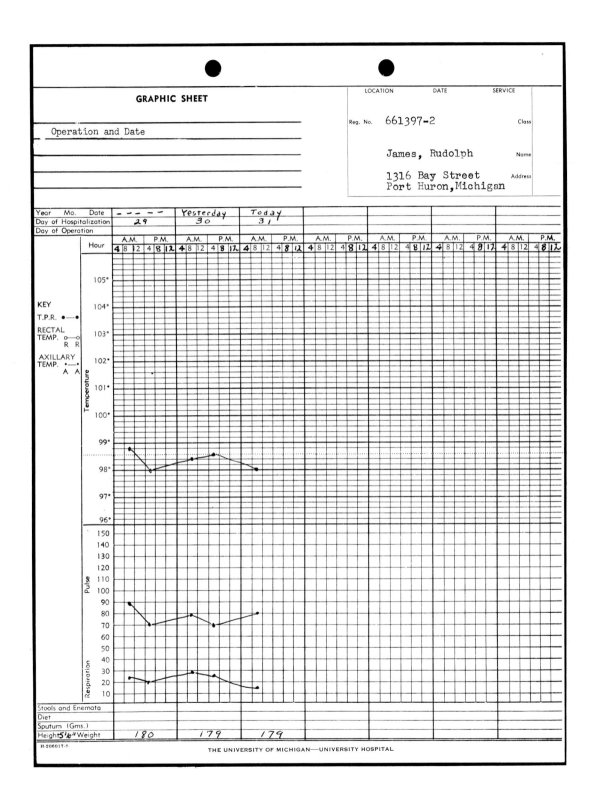

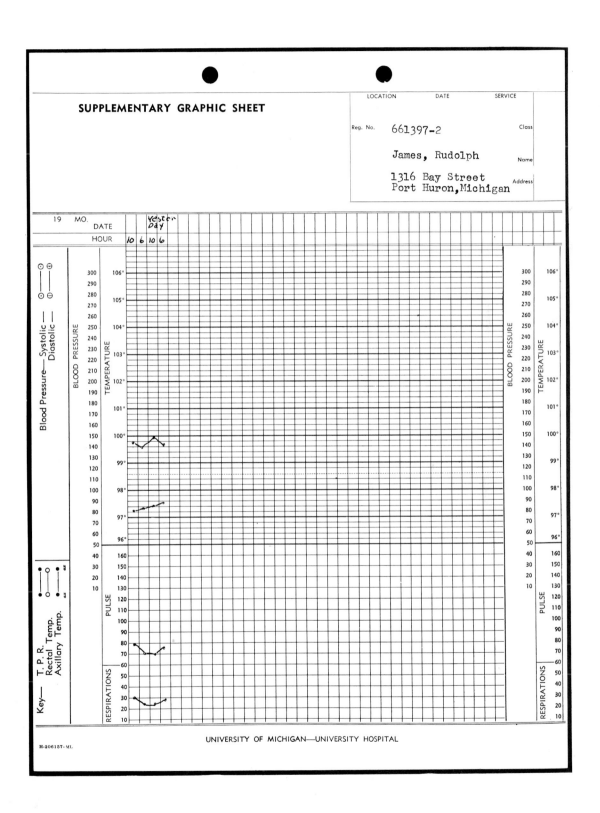

SUPPLEMENTARY GRAPHIC SHEET

LOCATION   DATE   SERVICE

Reg. No.   661397-2   Class

James, Rudolph   Name

1316 Bay Street   Address
Port Huron, Michigan

UNIVERSITY OF MICHIGAN—UNIVERSITY HOSPITAL

H-206157-ML

	LOCATION	DATE	SERVICE

INTAKE AND OUTPUT

TOTAL SHEET

Reg. No. 661397-2   Class

James, Rudolph   Name

1316 Bay Street   Address
Port Huron, Michigan

YR. MO. DATE	Yesterday			Today								
DAY OF HOSP.												
DAY OF OPERATION												
	8 A.M. 4 P.M.	4 P.M. 12 A.M.	12 A.M. 8 A.M.	8 A.M. 4 P.M.	4 P.M. 12 A.M.	12 A.M. 8 A.M.	8 A.M. 4 P.M.	4 P.M. 12 A.M.	12 A.M. 8 A.M.	8 A.M. 4 P.M.	4 P.M. 12 A.M.	12 A.M. 8 A.M.
INTAKE												
ORAL												
FORMULA												
INTRAVENOUS												
8 HOUR TOTAL	1230	440	100									
24 HOUR TOTAL	XXXXXXXXXXXXXX		1770	XXXXXXXXXXXXXX			XXXXXXXXXXXXX			XXXXXXXXXXXXX		
OUTPUT												
URINARY												
8 HOUR TOTAL	530	470	150									
24 HOUR TOTAL	XXXXXXXXXXXXXX		1150	XXXXXXXXXXXXXX			XXXXXXXXXXXXX			XXXXXXXXXXXXX		
NON-URINARY												
EMESIS												
WANGENSTEEN												
BILE												
THORACOTOMY												
8 HOUR TOTAL												
24 HOUR TOTAL	XXXXXXXXXXXXXX			XXXXXXXXXXXXXX			XXXXXXXXXXXXX			XXXXXXXXXXXXX		

H-206063-ML   THE UNIVERSITY OF MICHIGAN—UNIVERSITY HOSPITAL

MEDICATION RECORD

1. Routine medications—begin at top of sheet.
2. PRN and stat medications and infusions—begin at bottom of sheet. Record all infusion solutions and added medications.
3. Medications given—write hour in appropriate column.
4. Medications omitted—write hour in appropriate column and circle hour. Note reason on blue notes.
5. Medications discontinued—write "Discontinued" following time of last dosage given.
6. Changes in orders—discontinue first order.
7. Sign full name for each tour of duty.

LOCATION	DATE	SERVICE

REG. NO. 661397-2   CLASS

James, Rudolph   NAME

1316 Bay Street   ADDRESS
Port Huron, Michigan

MEDICATION ORDER				DATE Yesterday		DATE Today		DATE		FOR PHARMACY USE ONLY
				HOUR GIVEN		HOUR GIVEN		HOUR GIVEN		
DRUG	DOSAGE	ROUTE	FREQ	AM	PM	AM	PM	AM	PM	
Colace 100 mgm (o) q.d.				10						
Digitoxin 0.1mgm (o) q.d				10						
Seconal 100 mgm (o) hs. prn						9³⁰	1⁰⁰			

SIGNATURE	12:05 — 8:05 P. Ross	4:35 — 12:05 M. Nichols	12:05 — 8:05 P. Ross	4:35 — 12:05	12:05 — 8:05	4:35 — 12:05	
	8:05 — 1:05 J. Lewis	1:05 — 4:35	8:05 — 1:05	1:05 — 4:35	8:05 — 1:05	1:05 — 4:35	

H206189   THE UNIVERSITY OF MICHIGAN—UNIVERSITY HOSPITAL

BLUE COPY – MEDICAL RECORD

NURSING NOTES

1. Routines of care—write treatments and frequency; fill in time upon completion.
2. P.R.N. routines—write treatments and frequency, fill in time upon completion.
3. Write "AM" and "PM" midnite and noon only.
4. Leave two lines between routines and observations.
5. Write special tests or treatments and time completed above observations.
6. Write observations across full line.
7. Sign full name for each tour of duty.

LOCATION	DATE	SERVICE
Reg. No. 661397-2		Class

James, Rudolph   Name

1316 Bay Street   Address
Port Huron, Michigan

HOUR	OBSERVATION	TREATMENT

Yesterday

8-4 Pt. up in chair for 20" both morning and afternoon.
Stated that he did not feel tired after sitting. Pt.
is eating well and in good spirits.   J. Lewis

4-12 Quiet evening. Pt. up in chair for 20" x 1. Stated
that he felt slightly tired after he returned
to bed.   M. Nichols

Today

12-8 Awoke at 1 A.M., asked for repeat sleeping med.
Then slept through night.
P. Ross

THE UNIVERSITY OF MICHIGAN—UNIVERSITY HOSPITAL

LOCATION	NAME		SERVICE	AGE
10	Wicker, Gloria		E & M	55

EXP. DATE	STANDING MEDICATIONS	EXP. DATE	P. R. N. MEDICATIONS
3-16	Orinase 500 mgm. (o) q.d. (10ᴬ)	3-16	Darvon Cpd. 65 mgm.
3-16	Therapeutic multivits		(o) q 4° prn pain
	tab - ⊤ (o) q.d. (10ᴬ)	3-16	Seconal 100 mgm (o)
✓	Insulin look for dosage		h.s prn May repeat x1

ACME VISIBLE INDEX SYSTEM #84598-A

PRIVILEGES AND PRECAUTIONS:	TREATMENTS:
	Warm sterile saline soak to ulcer
Bed rest ⊂	Ⓛ ankle for 20' qid. (6ᴬ, 10ᴬ, 2ᴾ, 6ᴾ)
BRP	
	↑ left lower leg on 2 pillows
	at all times
TPR q. 4°	

UNIVERSITY HOSPITAL - UNIVERSITY OF MICHIGAN

FORM 206007 4/63 10M REV. 6-59   NURSING CARE CARD

GUIDES TO NURSING MANAGEMENT:

OPERATION AND DATE

DIAGNOSIS *diabetes mellitus, infected ulcer on left ankle*

DIET *1200 Calories diabetic* | I | O | RELIGION *Prot.* | ADMITTING DATE *yesterday*

LOCATION *10* | NAME *Wicker, Gloria* | SERVICE *E & M.* | AGE *55*

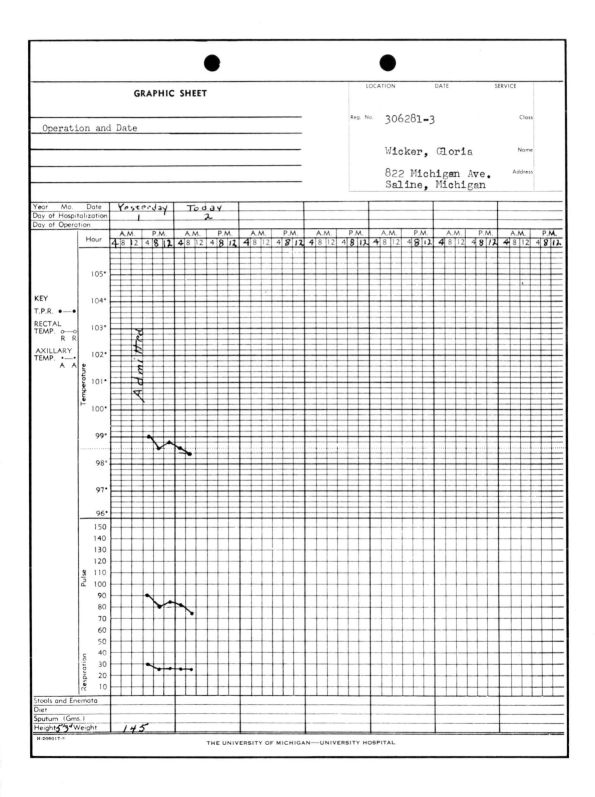

MEDICATION RECORD

1. Routine medications – begin at top of sheet.
2. P.R.N. and stat medications and infusions – begin at bottom of sheet. Record all infusion solutions and added medications.
3. Medications given – write hour in appropriate column.
4. Medications omitted – write hour in appropriate column and circle hour. Note reason on blue notes.
5. Medications discontinued – write "Discontinued" following time of last dosage given.
6. Changes in orders – discontinue first order.
7. Sign full name for each tour of duty.

LOCATION	DATE	SERVICE

REG. NO.   **306281-3**   CLASS

Wicker, Gloria (Mrs.) NAME

822 Michigan Ave.   ADDRESS
Saline, Michigan

MEDICATION ORDER				DATE Yesterday		DATE Today		DATE		FOR PHARMACY USE ONLY	
				HOUR GIVEN		HOUR GIVEN		HOUR GIVEN			
DRUG	DOSAGE	ROUTE	FREQ	AM	PM	AM	PM	AM	PM		
therapeutic multivita T (o)					2						
q d											
lente insulin						22 u /7$\frac{30}{}$					
Darvon Cpd. 65 mgm (o)				8$\frac{30}{}$		3					
q. 4° prn											
Seconal 100 mgm (o)				9 30		1 $\frac{30}{}$					
q h s prn											

SIGNATURE	12:05 — 8:05 P. Ross	4:35 — 12:05 M. Nichols	12:05 — 8:05 P.Ross	4:35 — 12:05	12:05 — 8:05	4:35 — 12:05	
	8:05 — 1:05	1:05 — 4:35 J. Lewis	8:05 — 1:05	1:05 — 4:35	8:05 — 1:05	1:05 — 4:35	

H206189   THE UNIVERSITY OF MICHIGAN – UNIVERSITY HOSPITAL

    BLUE COPY – MEDICAL RECORD

NURSING NOTES

1. Routines of care—write treatments and frequency; fill in time upon completion.
2. P.R.N. routines—write treatments and frequency, fill in time upon completion.
3. Write "AM" and "PM" midnite and noon only.
4. Leave two lines between routines and observations.
5. Write special tests or treatments and time completed above observations.
6. Write observations across full line.
7. Sign full name for each tour of duty.

LOCATION	DATE	SERVICE
Reg. No. 306281-3		Class
	Wicker, Gloria (Mrs.) Name	
	822 Michigan Ave. Address Saline, Michigan	

HOUR	OBSERVATION	TREATMENT

Yesterday

1 P.M. 55 year old white female admitted via wheelchair. Says she has "sore" on left ankle. Nurse observed open area size of 50 cent piece on outer aspect of left ankle: oozing purulent, greenish drainage c̄ small amount of bright red blood. Left foot edematous and purplish in color. Pt. appears to be in no acute pain. T 99 P 90 R 30. Urine specimen obtained

4 P.M. Resting in bed.   J. Lewis

4-12 Quiet evening. Seen by Dr. Wills. Pt. keeping leg elevated. Complains of dull ache in left ankle. Relieved somewhat by pain medication.   M. Nichols

Today

12-8 Slept at intervals. Repeat sleeping med. given at 1³⁵. Awake and complaining of pain in (L) ankle at 3 A.M. Pain medication given.
                         P. Ross

H-206025   THE UNIVERSITY OF MICHIGAN—UNIVERSITY HOSPITAL

Verbal Morning Report from Night Nurse: 8:00 A.M.

○ Mr. James is in bed 15. He got kind of tired after being up on the chair last evening, but felt all right once he returned to bed. He slept well last night. He only woke up at about 1:00 A.M. to ask for a repeat sleeping medication. His TPR is normal this morning. His vital signs last night were 142/86, P 74, and R 28. His intake and output totals from 8:00 A.M. yesterday until 8:00 A.M. today are I-1870 and O-1150. He has an appointment for a portable electrocardiogram at 10:00 A.M.

○ Mr. Cutler is in bed 5. He had a tough evening; his family was here for the evening and left about 9:00 P.M. When Mary Ann went in at 10:00 P.M. to get him ready for bed, he was crying. You know how well he's been doing since he had his left foot amputated two days ago? Well, I guess his family came and kept talking with him about how would he ever walk again, didn't his **leg** hurt, and how could they help him. They just kept going on and on and got him all wound up. Mary Ann gave him a sleeping med, but he was still awake when I came in. He got all upset again about 1:00 A.M. I tried to get him comfortable, gave him some pain medication, and finally he got to sleep. You know, it might help if the doctor were to talk with the family when they come again.

○ Mrs. Wicker is in bed 10. Were you here when she was admitted? Yes, well, she had a pretty quiet evening. She complained of pain in her left leg and had Darvon Compound last at 3:00 A.M. She also had some trouble sleeping and had a repeat sleeping med at 1:30 A.M. Her temperature is normal this morning. She keeps her leg elevated most of the time. She's to have a warm sterile soak to her left ankle this morning. This will be the first time she's had it.

Medical Information

Description of Preparation for Tests

Bronchogram
1. Permit to be obtained by physician.
2. Nothing by mouth 6 hours prior to appointment.
3. Seconal 100 mgm. orally and Demerol 50 mgm. (IM) 1 hour prior to x-ray appointment. Order to be written by physician.
4. Postural drainage for 15 minutes before appointment.
5. Patient to wear hospital gown, robe, and white socks.
6. Transportation: on stretcher.
7. Send patient's chart.

After Care
1. Nothing by mouth for 2 hours or until able to swallow.
2. Postural drainage stat upon return until bronchial tree is evacuated.
3. Urge to cough frequently.

Electrocardiogram (EKG)
1. Permit not required.
2. May eat prior to test.
3. Patient should rest for ½ hour prior to test.
4. Be sure patient has bath prior to test.
5. Wearing apparel: hospital gown.
6. Transportation: optional, according to patient's needs.

After Care
1. Remove electrode paste as soon as patient returns to unit.

Electromyogram (EMG)
1. On day of appointment
    a. Be sure patient has bath before test.
    b. On call medication: Demerol and Sparine. Order to be written by physician.
    c. Wearing apparel: hospital gown.
    d. Transportation: stretcher always, to Physical Medicine or Neurology Clinic as directed.

After Care
1. Check for needle site infections.

X-Ray
1. For chest and extremity x-ray, no special preparation is taken.

Diet Manual

GENERAL DIET

The general diet is planned to include these foods daily:

Milk	3 cups
Meat, fish, cheese, and legumes	3 ounces
Eggs	3-4 per week
Vegetable	2 servings other than potato, at least one green leafy or yellow and one raw
Fruit	2 servings, at least one good source of ascorbic acid
Bread or cereal	3 or more servings, whole grain or enriched
Butter	1 or more tablespoons

Additional foods, such as desserts, cream, nuts, jellies, dressings, sugar, gravy, etc., are given to make up the required calories.

LOW SODIUM DIET

(Approximately 800 mg. Sodium)

This diet is a general diet except that no salt, soda, or baking powder is used in the preparation of any food. (Salt substitutes without sodium are available for patients on this diet.) Because milk, eggs, meat, and fish are relatively high in sodium, they should not be served in larger than standard servings.

Beverage	Any kind, unsalted
Bread	Made without salt
Cereal	Any cooked without salt
	Puffed rice
	Puffed wheat
	Shredded wheat
Dessert	Cakes and cookies, unsalted
	Custard and pudding, from allowed foods
	Frozen dessert and ice cream, from allowed foods
	Gelatin dessert, from allowed foods
	Fruit whip, from allowed foods
	Pie, unsalted, from allowed foods
Fat	Any kind, unsalted
Fruit	Any kind
Meat	Unsalted meat, fish, poultry, cottage cheese, or eggs
Nuts	Any kind, unsalted
Potato or alternate	Any kind, unsalted
Seasoning	Any except salt or those containing salt or sodium
Soup	Cream, made from allowed foods
Sweets and flavorings	Any kind, unsalted
Vegetables	Any fresh, frozen, or canned without salt

Avoid . . . .
1. Salted, smoked, and prepared meats
2. Commercially frozen fish fillets and shellfish (except oysters)
3. Meat gravies and meat broths
4. Commercially canned vegetables, relishes, and salad dressings, except those prepared without salt or sodium
5. Any cheese, except unsalted cottage
6. Commercially frozen peas and lima beans
7. Quick cooking cereals, commercially prepared mixes

1200 CALORIE DIABETIC DIET

The diabetic diet is adapted to the nutritional needs of the individual patient and to his personal taste within available limits. Orders specify the grams of protein, grams of carbohydrate, and number of calories desired. Unless otherwise ordered, the carbohydrate is divided evenly among the three meals. 1200 cal: 70 grams protein, 45 grams fat, and 130 grams carbohydrate.

1. Total calories depend upon patients nutritional status and degree of activity.
2. Carbohydrate allowances vary roughly in accordance with total calories.
3. Protein allowances also vary with total calories.
4. Fat makes up the caloric difference after carbohydrate and protein calories have been determined.
5. The carbohydrate, protein, and fat should not vary more than 5 grams from the diet prescription. Calories should not vary more than 25. Division of carbohydrate among the meals should not vary more than 5 grams from 1/3 of calculated carbohydrate.
6. If food is refused, the carbohydrate (5 grams or more per meal or 10 grams per day) is replaced.
7. Foods with caloric value should not be added to the diet or substituted for other foods without the permission of the physician and consultation with a dietician. However, unsweetened tea and coffee may be given to the patient if he desires them and is not on fluid restrictions.

Medical-Nursing Textbook*

CONGESTIVE HEART FAILURE:

Causes of failure in the pumping mechanism of the heart can generally be labeled under 3 headings: (1) failure to fill, (2) overloading, and (3) deterioration in functional capacity. Manifestations of heart failure usually develop gradually. Signs and symptoms in congestive heart failure arise from the failure of the heart to adequately nourish and oxygenate the tissues and from the accumulation of blood and fluid in the various tissues and organs in the body. In the early stages of congestive heart failure the most outstanding symptom is shortness of breath during ordinary activities. The patient is frequently apprehensive and has less energy than before. Later on, pulmonary edema may develop, accompanied by dyspnea, Cheyne-Stokes respiration, cyanosis, and cough with blood tinged sputum. Finally, generalized systemic edema occurs with a fluid weight gain of 15 to 30 pounds, and because of this, the patient is more susceptible to developing decubiti. There is also involvement of the G.I. tract with the symptoms of anorexia, nausea, and vomiting.

Treatment is aimed at reestablishing the efficiency of the heart as a pump. This involves increasing the force or strength of the contraction of the myocardium and reducing the demands made on the myocardium until the efficiency of the pumping mechanism has been restored. Both aspects of treatment are carried out simultaneously. The physician prescribes a cardiac glucoside, usually a preparation of digitalis, to strengthen the force of cardiac contraction, a regime of rest and activity to limit the demands made on the failing heart; and diuretics combined with sodium restriction to reduce the volume of fluid in the body and thus lessen the burden on the weakened heart.

---

*From Beland, *Clinical Nursing.* New York: The Macmillan Co., 1965.

DIABETES MELLITUS:

Diabetes mellitus is a chronic hereditary disorder not only of carbohydrate metabolism but of fat, protein, electrolyte, and water metabolism as well. Authorities generally agree that the metabolic defects result from a relative or absolute lack of insulin. Early signs and symptoms of diabetes include increasing glucose levels in the blood and in the urine, thirst, increased urinary output, and increased appetite, often with weight loss and weakness. Diabetes mellitus also increases susceptibility to certain types of infections, particularly those of the skin. Complications resulting from diabetes include hypoglycemia and acidosis, reduced functioning of the kidneys, blindness due to cataracts and retinopathy, arthero-sclerosis, and vascular complications.

Successful control of diabetes depends upon the intelligent cooperation of the patient and his family. General objectives of medical therapy include:

1. Individualize the patient's regime so that he can live as full and useful a life as is possible within the limitations of his disorder.

2. To correct the underlying metabolic imbalance.

3. To attain and maintain ideal body weight.

4. To prevent or delay the onset and progression of complication of the disease.

The objectives of the therapy of diabetes are achieved by diet, insulin, education, and exercise. Since the diabetic is more susceptible to skin infections, he should take care to keep especially clean. His feet require special care: freedom from binding shoes and socks, cleanliness, and observation to see that there are no sore places which could break down since the diabetic may have arteriosclerosis and may not heal as rapidly as the more healthy individual. If ulcerations occur, pressure on that area should be avoided by keeping any unnecessary weight, such as bed clothes, off the area and by keeping the pressure of the body part off the area. Measures should also be taken to improve the circulation to that area by applying warm compress or elevating the body part. Extremities should be protected from pressure and from heat. The patient should eat the foods in his diet *in the amounts ordered,* since not adhering to his diet will upset his metabolic processes. Therefore, food substitutions or additions are not made without consulting the physician and the dietician, while the patient is in the hospital. The major responsibilities of the nurse to the diabetic patient are caring for him when he is ill and instructing the patient in the management of his condition.